Surgical Renaissance in the Heartland

Also by Henry Buchwald

———

Metabolic Surgery
with Richard Varco

Surgical Management of Obesity
with George Cowan Jr. and Walter Pories

Pioneers in Gastroenterology
with Walford Gillison

*Atlas of Metabolic and Bariatric Surgical Techniques
and Procedures*

Let Me Tell You a Story, Volumes I to III

Surgical Renaissance in the Heartland

A MEMOIR
of the
WANGENSTEEN ERA

Henry Buchwald

University of Minnesota Press
Minneapolis
London

This is a work of nonfiction. No names have been altered and no scenes have been invented. In my recollection of events, places, and people, I have not knowingly misstated or misquoted. I used direct quotations for what I heard, and I paraphrased reliable witnesses when applicable in my best effort to be accurate.

Copyright 2020 by Henry Buchwald

Published by the University of Minnesota Press
111 Third Avenue South, Suite 290
Minneapolis, MN 55401-2520
http://www.upress.umn.edu

Printed in the United States of America on acid-free paper

The University of Minnesota is an equal-opportunity educator and employer.

25 24 23 22 21 20   10 9 8 7 6 5 4 3 2 1

Library of Congress Cataloging-in-Publication Data
Buchwald, Henry, author.
Surgical renaissance in the heartland : a memoir of the Wangensteen era / Henry Buchwald.
LCCN 2019027052 (print) | ISBN 978-1-5179-1011-2 (hc) | ISBN 978-1-5179-0994-9 (pb)
Subjects: LCSH: Buchwald, Henry. | Wangensteen, Owen H. (Owen Harding), 1898–1981. | University of Minnesota. Department of Surgery—History—20th century. | Surgeons—United States—Biography.
Classification: LCC RD27.35.B836 A3 2020 (print) | DDC 617.092 [B]—dc23
LC record available at https://lccn.loc.gov/2019027052

*I dedicate this book to the person who has made my life,
Daisy Emilie, now my wife of sixty-five years. She gave me the
inspiration for my career and supported me in my ambitions.
Her love is unconditional, as is mine for her.*

*I dedicate this book to my children—Dana, Claire and Larry,
Amy and Danny, and Jane and Tim,
and to my grandchildren—Catherine, Alexander, Rose, Sarah,
Eden, and Trevor, who inspire and encourage me.*

*To my many coworkers and friends,
I say thank you for our years together.*

*And to my parents, who gave me life, saved me from death,
provided me with sustenance, and watched over me with
curiosity and approbation, an everlasting thank you.*

Contents

Prologue . . . ix

1. Beginnings . . . 1

2. The Roots of the Wangensteen Era . . . 17

3. Settling into Minnesota . . . 34

4. Culture Shock . . . 44

5. Anoka and Stillwater . . . 52

6. Wangensteen's Surgery Service . . . 62

7. Early Research . . . 75

8. Varco's Surgery Service . . . 82

9. Laboratory Founded . . . 92

10. Laboratory Funded . . . 105

11. Senior Resident . . . 117

12. Colleagues . . . 125

13. Chief Resident . . . 133

14. Assistant Professor . . . 146

15. Endgame . . . 153

Epilogue . . . 170

Acknowledgments . . . 183

Index . . . 185

Prologue

Have I raised the next generation?

————

THE TALMUD, Tractate Shabbat

This is a personal memoir of a golden era in American surgery, of a department of surgery in a medical school in Minnesota, flyover land to many Easterners. These were years that forever changed medicine and the lives of millions.

Surgery was a limited discipline until the advent of anesthesia and antisepsis in the nineteenth century. From then until the mid-twentieth century, the domain of surgery expanded markedly to encompass massive resectional procedures, transplantation, and complex reparative surgery. This heady and universal growth of surgery in these disciplines, as well as operative innovations, often emanated from the University of Minnesota in the United States heartland. The foundations of surgery for bowel obstruction, obesity, open-heart procedures, heart transplantation, pancreas transplants for diabetes, intestinal bypass for elevated cholesterol levels, implantable infusion pump therapies, and other landmark procedures originated here. Owen H. Wangensteen, son of a Minnesota farmer, initiated this ferment of productivity. His protégés— Richard Varco, the Lillehei brothers Walton and Richard, and many others who will long be remembered in the annals of medicine— also did not come from the Eastern establishment but were independent spirits from the Midwest and the West. Wangensteen's creation of a singular residency training program designed to graduate academic surgeons dedicated to solving real-life problems through research served as a cauldron for thought, experiment, and implementation.

This book explores the roots, heritage, and traditions underlying the unique contributions of the University of Minnesota Department of Surgery to medicine and to the lives of those reading this volume. My own professional and personal life intersected with this history in the culminating years of the Minnesota dynasty and continued after the Wangensteen era through the later lives of the main actors in this real-life drama.

I tell this story from my perspective because I lived it. I knew the people. I know the events that took place. Others would tell this story differently, with different events, anecdotes, and insights into the lives of the surgeons of that epoch. For that reason, I have also written extensively of my life prior to arriving in Minnesota. My vision and reflections are those of an American born in Austria, a child of the Holocaust, a Midwesterner from the East—imbued (or perhaps afflicted) with the outlook, sense of humor, and spirit of independence that often seem to accompany the surgical personality.

This retrospective of a particular past will, I hope, offer insights pertinent to the future.

Surgical Renaissance in the Heartland

✴ 1 ✴

Beginnings

> The Practice of Medicine is an art,
> not a trade; a calling, not a business;
> a calling in which your heart will be
> exercised equally with your head.
>
> ──────
> WILLIAM OSLER, *Aequanimitas:*
> *The Master-word in Medicine*, 1914

We drove to Minneapolis that first day in a mini-caravan, I in my recently acquired black, English Ford Popular with a right-hand drive, floor stick shift, a nonfunctioning heater, and a hand crank for those times when the starter would not work. I was followed by Daisy Emilie, my wife, in our blue Ford sedan. Both cars were packed with our personal possessions, with our sparse furniture to follow. In Daisy's care, tucked into her car seat, rode our first child, Jane, age two.

Earlier that day—September 11, 1960—I was honored, surprised, and astonished in that order; my mood was nostalgic. It was my last day as Chief Flight Surgeon, Strategic Air Command, U.S. Air Force, stationed at SAC headquarters, Offutt Air Force Base, outside of Bellevue, Nebraska, a small town near Omaha. It was also my first official day in the Department of Surgery of the Medical School of the University of Minnesota.

On the morning of our departure, I went to my office for the

I

last time. My staff had already given me a farewell party, and I had previously packed the model SAC planes I had received as gifts. I came to sort personal papers and belongings and to leave a note of welcome for my replacement. After less than an hour, I was ready to depart. As I opened my office door, I saw my staff, in their dress blue uniforms rather than their usual white hospital attire, lined up along the corridor to my office. Sergeant West, the office NCOIC (Non-Commissioned Officer in Charge), barked, "Attention, commanding officer relinquishing command." They all saluted. I worked my way down the line, shaking hands amid mutual words of good luck. This departure ceremony was not prescribed and I had not expected it. That event remains one of my fondest memories of my time in the Air Force as a flight surgeon.

I walked to headquarters to pick up my final orders at the office of the personnel colonel who had given me my introductory SAC lecture. The orders were waiting for me in a sealed envelope. When I made my farewells, the colonel looked as if he were expecting me to say something more than good-bye. I told him that it had been both a great honor and a pleasure to have served in SAC. He gave me an inscrutable smile, which puzzled me. As I walked to my car, though still in uniform, I felt like a civilian in a world I was no longer part of.

When I reached the car, I opened my orders. I wanted to read the phrase "Honorable Discharge." Instead, I read, "Extended Active Duty, Subject to Immediate Recall." I raced back to the personnel office. The colonel said, "I thought you would be back." I told him that my assignment to SAC headquarters had been mysterious to me, but that my departure orders were even more so. I held them up and inquired what they meant. He responded that the orders were so issued because I had top-secret clearance, I had been at SAC headquarters command, SAC had the authority to retain me, and SAC had done so. Therefore, until the age of forty, I would have to undergo and submit the results of an annual flight physical and electrocardiogram, inform SAC headquarters where I resided, and be subject to being summoned by a telephone call to report immediately for active duty in SAC. Several years later, when the war in Vietnam broke out, I was expecting that call. It never came. The generals on the staff of SAC I had come to know had moved on, and SAC itself was evolving into a new elite command, combined with the Navy SEALs, Delta Force, Army Rangers, and other rapid-strike units, collectively referred to as Special Operations Command. I was easy to replace. Fortunately, this country will always have capable young men and women to take their turn in the armed forces of our nation. My Air Force interlude left an indelible memory, a time in my life in which I take great pride and that in many ways has shaped my thinking.

I had always known that I needed to find a surgical training program to enter when my Air Force tour was completed. Although Daisy and my parents hoped that we would return to New York, I was not eager to do so. The eastern surgery residencies were limited to clinical training, with little or no opportunity for research. They were also structured as competitive pyramids where only some of those who started in the program finished as a chief resident. I had encountered more than I wanted of this kind of peer competition for advancement based on the opinion of others. I was ready to compete on the basis of my clinical competence and to do some real work in basic research. Further, I had marked my time at Columbia University's College of Physicians and Surgeons (P&S) by several acts interpretable as insubordination. For example, prior to my departure from my internship, I had called the pompous chief resident "an insolent, arrogant puppy."

During my time at SAC, I had heard of the unique surgery training program at the University of Minnesota under Owen H. Wangensteen, a program for individuals planning an academic career that incorporated several years of research into an extended residency. I made an appointment in the spring of 1960 for an interview at the University of Minnesota and at the world-famous Mayo Clinic in Rochester, Minnesota, fifty miles south of the Twin Cities of Minneapolis and St. Paul.

I visited the Mayo Clinic first. Although I found the program impressive, it did not include the research opportunities I was seeking. I drove to Minneapolis and spent the afternoon at the University of Minnesota, located in the rapidly growing city of Minneapolis. The University of Minnesota had (and has) the largest dedicated population of students, faculty, and staff at a single campus in the United States. Within this campus complex, straddling the Mississippi River and situated on a bluff on the east side of the river, was the University Hospital and Medical School. Starting from humble beginnings less than a generation earlier, by the 1950s the Department of Surgery was extremely large and employed well over twenty residents on the clinical services and probably more than an equal number in departmental laboratories or studying for PhD degrees in the basic sciences. The residents I talked to were happy with their choice of a training program and were focused on making a research contribution in an academic setting. They were living my medical school dream. It was not, after all, a phantasm. This opportunity actually existed in the middle of the great northern prairie.

In the late afternoon, I had my interview with the chair of surgery, Dr. Owen H. Wangensteen. He was a trim man of relatively short stature, energetic in his movements. He appeared to be a man used to physical work. I later learned that he grew up on a Minnesota farm, the son of Norwegian farmers. When asked why he had chosen to be a surgeon, his stock response was that "It beat milking cows at 5 o'clock in the morning." Behind his glasses, his eyes had a perpetual look of amusement. He spoke in a rather high-pitched voice with a flawless command of the English language. As I learned over time, he thought and spoke in paragraphs rather than in phrases or sentences; he exuded knowledge and was intolerant of wasted time. Contrary to my experience with the faculties of the Ivy League medical schools, his questioning was not about my background, my race, religion, money, and potential influence, but about my seriousness of purpose and my desire for learning. He was interested in my aspirations and in my prior research experience as a medical student. He told me that his program involved a minimum of seven years: the usual four years of clinical residency subsequent to a one-year internship, and at least two years in the laboratory. I must have literally jumped at the idea or at least responded with joy when he offered me a job. I accepted. These were the days before the national, electronic residency match of the choices of applicants and academic institutions.

I returned to Offutt Air Force Base and made my intentions to return to a civilian surgical training program known. I must have done something right during my tenure at Offutt because several of the senior officers attempted to keep me in the Air Force and in SAC. I was given three tempting choices to sign on for retention: moving to NASA to compete with selected flight surgeons from the other branches of the armed services to be the first doctor in space; electing a prized two-year duty assignment overseas; or taking senior flight surgeon status and promotion from my rank as captain after two years spent at the Harvard School of Public Health where I would obtain a PhD. All of these options, however, led to a pensioned dead end at a fairly young age. Most important, they did not lead to a career in surgery, my choice for the way I wished to spend my working life.

Why did I choose surgery? The answer lies in the story of my past.

I was born on June 21, 1932, in the Rudolphina House Hospital in Vienna, Austria. The following year, the first Nazi concentration camp opened in the German town of Dachau, close to Munich, ignored by most of the world. Hitler and Nazi Germany had determined that Jews, Gypsies, homosexuals, and other groups should be arrested, taken out of society, and incarcerated in overcrowded labor and starvation camps, on the path to an organized system of extermination, of genocide. The governments of the democratic societies, including those of France, Great Britain, and the United States, stood back and pretended not to notice.

Jews were the primary genocidal target of Nazi Germany–conquered Europe. Eventually, most of European Jewry, numbering more than six million men, women, and children, were annihilated. The largest concentration of Jews in the world at that time was tortured, gassed, shot, reduced to ashes, and relegated to mass graves. And the governments of the World War II Allies clearly indicated that millions of these hardworking, productive human souls, and their unborn prodigy, were not on their nations' moral compass. The shocking, cold-blooded extinction of Jews did not raise an ethical outcry. This silence of Holocaust bystanders is one of humanity's greatest examples of moral turpitude.

In 1944, the Nazi concentration camp killing of Jews had moved into high gear, increasing in volume and efficiency. Yet even Hitler was not quite certain of the response of the Allies to his policy of mass murder. He, via Adolf Eichmann, offered the Allies a trade of one million Hungarian Jews for ten thousand trucks—one hundred lives for one truck. Roosevelt and Great Britain refused. Hitler's realization that the extermination of Jews would not trouble other world leaders was confirmed. To fulfill the final solution for the Jews, Eichmann organized the transfer of these Hungarian Jews to concentration camps in Poland and in Germany, from which few emerged at the end of the war. Some of the family from my Hungarian roots survived the war and were swallowed up in the postwar dominance of Hungary by the Soviet Union.

By 1944, the tide of war in Europe was turning. The Allies were seeing progress on the western front, and the Soviet Union was winning on the eastern front. During this time of growing hope and overwhelming resources, Jewish groups and Jewish refugees were sending emissary after emissary to the West Wing of the White House and, at times, gaining an audience with President Roosevelt. They pleaded with the U.S. government to bomb the railheads leading to the concentration camps in order to hinder the flow of European Jewry to annihilation. They even asked that the concentration camps be bombed, and, at the cost of Jewish lives, be put out of action. At the same time, Stalin, head of the Soviet Union, requested that these bombings *not* take place, for if they were successful, German forces—in particular the elite SS troops, as well as German transportation—might be diverted to the Russian front. The governments of the Allied nations, notably the United States, which had by this time undisputed air supremacy in Europe, did not bomb the railheads and tracks or the concentration camps. Although this may have been a valid strategic decision, I will never condone it.

In 1938, my father was arrested, his photo shop in Vienna destroyed, and his inventory looted. He was miraculously saved from a concentration camp by a Nazi commandant, who, like my father, was an Austrian-Hungarian army veteran of World War I. That man warned my father that Jewish former officers with my father's record of valor and commendations would be among the first to be annihilated. That night, my father made plans for us to emigrate to the United States, where his sister and mother had previously taken residence, and where his American uncle and cousins had become established citizens in New York City prior to the turn of the twentieth century.

My father first met his American cousins during World War I when, through Red Cross channels, they agreed to meet on furlough in Switzerland. My father's cousins were with the American Expeditionary Forces, under General John J. Pershing in France, and my father was on the Italian front. They were relieved to learn from one another that they would not be exposed to opposing action. Our cousins promptly issued the request for visas. They were granted for my mother and for me but not for my father. By birth, my father was Hungarian; my mother and I were Austrian. The U.S. government, under Franklin D. Roosevelt, refused, in this time of persecution and genocide, to drop the quota system, and Hungarians were considered less desirable than Austrians. Not that Austrian or German Jews were given much better consideration; the United States granted only 27,370 visas to Jews from Austria and Germany and left three hundred thousand on an unfulfilled waiting list.

At first, my mother refused to leave without my father. They had been happily married for nine years. He persuaded her, however, to leave for my sake as well as her own. He convinced her that if we were safely out of Austria, he could flee to his native Hungary where he stood a much better chance of survival alone. And it was true—the good Christian people of the village in which he grew up risked their own lives, the lives of their children, their farms and possessions, to give him sanctuary. Possibly, the villagers remembered my father's parents, who ran the only general store, the focal point of the village, and when times were bad provided credit or accepted payment in eggs, cheese, bread, or, when it was available, meat. Perhaps the villagers remembered my father's uncle, the local veterinarian, who came when summoned, in summer or in winter, in all kinds of weather, whenever an animal was sick. The villagers moved my father at night from farm to farm. They fed him. He slept in attics and stables. In this manner, they hid him for nearly a year until, in 1939, he received his visa and was one of the last to be allowed to leave Nazi Europe.

In Vienna, we lived with my maternal grandparents, whom I remember ever so fondly. My grandmother was terminally ill, and my grandfather, a biochemist who was refused a university post because he would not convert to Christianity, remained at her side and buried her in a double grave with her sister. He wrote us that he was fleeing to Poland, the country of his birth, to join the Jewish partisans. In his sixties, he was physically strong. We never heard how long he survived. I do not know when he died, where he died, or how he died.

This was the world of my birth and early youth; the world of an Austrian-born Jew who would make the United States home and country, and who had just completed two years in the service of that country. Ironically, I was going to make my family's home in Minneapolis, which, in 1960, was known (but unbeknown to me) as the anti-Semitic capital of the United States.

In the United States, we lived first with my paternal grandmother and my aunt in a small apartment in Harlem in New York City. I was six years old when I arrived, and the first English-language instruction I received was on the streets. We subsequently moved to Sheepshead Bay, a fishing village on Long Island where the commercial fishing boats came in with their catch of cod, bluefish, and tuna for the big city. There we lived with a maternal aunt who had immigrated to the United States several years earlier. She was a milliner who made ladies' hats. My mother did piecework at home, gluing feathers and the like onto greeting cards, for a penny a card.

We arrived too late in the fall of that year for me to start school. My English was hardly sufficient for first grade or even for kindergarten. I believe the school officials of Sheepshead Bay had no knowledge of my existence. For months I roamed the streets, particularly the docks. I asked the fishermen if I could help them unload.

Some of them laughed at my size, or at my Germanic English. Over time, I broadened my vocabulary with the seamen's colorful language. They invited me to explore their boats and allowed me to help unloading fish or arranging them on the dock. When a boat was nearly empty, the fisherman would pick one or two good-looking fish and give them to me. I brought home dinner almost nightly. I told my mother and my aunt that the fishermen gave me the fish, which they did. I did not tell them that I worked many hours for my wages. I worked hard, I contributed to the household, and I was very proud. I could not as yet read. I had not read the paeans lauding the land of opportunity, but I firmly believed that I now lived in this land of opportunity.

When my father arrived in the United States, he entered the jewelry business, his occupation prior to his work at the Vienna photo store. We moved to a ground-floor apartment with barred windows in Flatbush, the toughest Brooklyn neighborhood in the toughest borough of New York City. My English now took on the patois of the city. I could not read or write. I was illiterate in two languages. I started school one year older than my peers. After school, I earned my PhD in survival with my fists.

In 1942, we moved to a second-floor apartment in a five-story walk-up, in the Inwood section of upper Manhattan, populated by hardworking people of mixed ethnicity. I was placed in the "hopeless" class of public school, where barely any attempt was made at education. And then an angel came into my life in the person of Mrs. Feil, a teacher with the power of deciding the fate of students. She saw some intellectual potential in me and moved me from the "five" class to the "opportunity" class—from the bottom rung to the top. There I fell in with a group of seven boys. We called ourselves the "Wolf Pack." These boys were smart, read outside of our studies, and listened to classical music. Interestingly, they were all athletic

and ignited the spark of athleticism in me that has provided me
happiness all my life.

I have rarely met a surgeon for whom sports or some kind of
physical activity was not an essential part of life. I played softball
and basketball during my time in public school, played varsity
soccer in high school and semiprofessional soccer on weekends. I
swam on the varsity team in college and played tennis. As an adult
later in life I took up skiing, marathon running, and working out
in a gymnasium.

From junior high school, I went on to the Bronx High School of
Science, a competitive magnet school, and subsequently to Columbia College. I chose to enter the College of Physicians and Surgeons
of Columbia University on professional option after my third year
of college, returning to graduate with my college class of '54 as
class valedictorian. Those were years of growth and education in
school and out of school. To earn my books, travel, and other living
expenses, I worked when not in school, in order to be a full-time
student on full-tuition scholarships in both college and medical
school. During spring and fall intersessions and during Christmas
vacation, I found employment as a mail carrier, a garment-district
shipping clerk, a soda-bottling assembly worker and truck loader,
and road construction laborer. I also worked as a vat mixer, making
a high-caloric patented formula to promote weight gain. During
the summer proper, I lifeguarded or worked as a senior boys' counselor in an athletic camp.

On June 6, 1954, Daisy Emilie Bix gave me the honor of becoming Mrs. Buchwald. We had known each other for five years, introduced by our parents when Daisy was fourteen and I was seventeen.
Our parents had rented summer cottages on the same street in a
little town in the Catskill Mountains. I was lifeguarding in a hotel
in a neighboring town but slept in a small hut next to my parents'

house to avoid sharing a room with a tuberculous dishwasher at the hotel.

Our engagement and marriage were in conflict with the mores of the time. We were considered too young to marry. Daisy was admitted to Barnard College of Columbia University on a full-tuition scholarship while I was in my first year at P&S. Both Daisy's freshman counselor and her freshman English professor tried, unsuccessfully, to convince her not to marry in June of her freshman year. But Daisy was unconvinced and so she became Barnard's first married student.

I was, as it happens, denied an internship because of my marriage. I was at the top of my medical school class. I believed that I had a good chance to choose where I would go for my internship, and I wanted the prestige of a Harvard internship. I spent a morning visiting and being interviewed at the Massachusetts General Hospital and the afternoon at the Peter Bent Brigham. At the Mass General, I was interviewed by the chairman of the department of surgery, Dr. Dwight Harken. He was not at all friendly. Looking at me critically, he started the interview by asking, "Do you really believe you would be comfortable here?" I knew then and there that a surgical internship at the Mass General was out of the question. I answered, "Oh, yes sir, having spent the morning here, I already feel six feet tall and blond." He frowned and responded, "What kind of a name is Buchwald?" In German, Buchwald means beech wood. There are as many German, Austrian, and Hungarian Catholic "Beechwoods" as Jewish ones. I was not going to give him the answer he was looking for. Instead, I provided him with a detailed history of the town of Hercegszöllős, my father's birthplace. That response ended my interview.

My interview went much better at the Peter Bent Brigham. I was shown around by the house staff and then had the good fortune to join rounds with the great Dr. Francis (Franny) Moore, chairman of the Department of Surgery. I liked him, and I believe he liked me. In our interview, it was obvious that he had carefully read my transcript and recommendations. He noted that I had signed the "no skiing" agreement. That was easy. At that time, I had never skied. After some pleasant banter, he looked at me and stated, "We have a problem." Because he was straightforward and blunt, I believed he would raise the Jewish question. But instead of saying, "We have never had a Jewish intern" (which was true), he said, "We have never had a married intern." He continued, "I am willing to make an exception. We require our interns to live in the quadrangle and spend their free time there with the other members of the house staff, since the camaraderie of the training experience is extremely important. The no-married-interns rule is a long-standing Brigham tradition. I suggest you accept the post and leave your wife in New York; I will turn a blind eye to your going to see her once a month." I thanked Dr. Moore but said that my marriage was predicated on togetherness. Because my wife had been accepted to the graduate school at Radcliffe, and because there was no vacation during the surgical internship (interns worked and slept at the hospital every other night at all institutions), I asked him if he could see his way to allowing me to rent an apartment in Boston, where I could stay on the two or three nights a week when I was not on call. He said he could not bend the rules, and so we parted. Interestingly, years later we became friends, and he invited me to be a visiting professor at the Brigham.

Daisy turned down Radcliffe and accepted the fellowship offered her at Columbia to study for her MA degree. Previously she had received her BA from Barnard College; she subsequently earned her PhD plus an honorary doctorate from the University of Minnesota. She is a writer, with four books to her credit, and became a renowned editor and publisher.

I accepted the proffered internship in the Department of Surgery at the Columbia-Presbyterian Medical Center. At Presbyterian I met Jack Bloch, who was to become a close friend until his death many years later. We were the only Jews on the surgical service, breaking an institutional precedent. We felt no discrimination, except for the annual house staff Christmas party at the home of the chair, Dr. George H. Humphreys II. His feast traditionally featured pork. Neither Jack nor I kept the kosher dietary laws, but I refused to eat pig that night on principle.

At the beginning of medical school, I had not decided in what area of medicine I would practice. I enjoyed every course I took in college and medical school. I was fascinated by the insect vectors in public health, I liked the intricacies of biochemistry, and, certainly, I enjoyed the intellectual stimulation of internal medicine. I was less impressed by the teaching and noncognitive focus of surgery at P&S. I took my third-year summer externship at the Mary Imogene Bassett Hospital in Cooperstown, New York, where I met and admired a technically superb and intellectually stimulating faculty who had chosen to come to this community hospital from Harvard, Columbia, and Johns Hopkins. The chief of surgery was Dr. John H. Powers. He was an extremely competent technical surgeon, a scholar, and a dedicated teacher.

A favorite saying of his was, "The knife falls at seven." Indeed, the knife fell at 7 o'clock every morning in every operating room at the Mary Imogene Bassett Hospital. The rule of silence prevailed in the operating room, except for Dr. Powers's teaching, which started either with his questioning the chief resident and working his way down to me, or with me and ascending to the chief resident.

After dinner on one of the last evenings in Cooperstown, Daisy and I walked down to the dock on Lake Otsego, close to the cabin we had rented for the summer. On that quiet night, the moonlight outshone the stars and was reflected in the water. This, however,

was not a night for romance. I had to make a decision. Was I going
to be a surgeon or an internist?

We made lists of the pros and cons for each choice. Internal
medicine was the premier department at P&S. The internists, as a
body, were the most knowledgeable, respected, and powerful physicians at that institution. Dr. Robert Loeb, chair of the Department of Medicine, had offered me a highly coveted internship in
medicine at P&S. In contradistinction, surgery was considered a
mechanical adjunct to medical therapy. I knew of no surgeon at
Columbia engaged in basic research. Rational thought and our list-
ing of advantages and disadvantages, therefore, strongly favored the
choice of internal medicine. Yet, I yearned for a training program,
an academic environment and institution for intellectual surgeons,
where a surgeon could operate, competently care for the nonsurgical problems of his patients, conduct basic research, teach, and be
an intellectual contributor to medical progress, and possibly even
be a scholar. At that time, I had not heard of the University of Minnesota, Owen H. Wangensteen, his staff, or his training program. I
had no knowledge that my dream actually existed.

I asked Daisy what I should do. Her response was short and
definitive: "Follow your heart." Without hesitation, I stated that my
heart chose surgery. Did I select surgery, or did surgery select me?
Who knows? What I knew on that dock that night in Cooperstown
was that surgery fit me like a surgical glove. I have never regretted
my decision.

I had made one other trip to Minneapolis before our journey
on September 11, 1960, the start of our lives as Minnesotans. In July
of that year, I took Daisy and Jane to see their future home. We
entered Minneapolis near the Foshay Tower, at the time the only
moderately tall building in the city. On our arrival, we noticed a
great commotion on a main street of the city, Nicollet Avenue.

I drove closer to the sound of marching bands. Soon we found ourselves part of a parade, which we had somehow blundered into. A policeman ordered us off to a side street. We told him that we were strangers to the city. Instead of giving us a ticket, he found us a restricted area where we could park our car. He told us to enjoy the annual Aquatennial Parade. We were introduced to "Minnesota Nice."

The Roots of the Wangensteen Era

> *When a sick cow, horse, or pig*
> *presented itself, my father called the*
> *veterinarian. In those days he usually*
> *would say that the only thing to do*
> *was either to let nature take its course*
> *or to terminate the situation by a blow*
> *on the head, by which suggestion I*
> *could not agree.*

OWEN H. WANGENSTEEN, *Surgery*
Clinics of North America, 1967

All the trees in a grove of aspens are interconnected by one root system. Whether they are adult trees or juveniles, they are a colony with a uniform and singular identity. While each tree can live the length of a human lifespan, such a grove of trees can live for thousands of years. Even if a single tree falls or is destroyed by fire, the common entity continues. The intertwined aspen root system is in constant communication and will add new offshoots to perpetuate its heritage. The roots are rhizogenic in nature, meaning that their large clonal clusters derive their origin from a single seedling. That seedling, for the University of Minnesota surgery department, was Owen H. Wangensteen.

Owen Harding Wangensteen was born in 1898 to Ove and

Hannah, of Norwegian ancestry, in the hamlet of Lake Park, Minnesota. Owen's mother died when he was seven. His father raised Owen, his two brothers, and one sister. Ove stressed education to his children, though Owen and his siblings were needed to help run the family farm. To these chores Owen contributed more than his brothers. He is quoted as saying on several occasions, "They learned to hunt, but I learned to work. And I think I got the best of the deal."

During Owen's junior year in high school, the family herd of fifty sows was unable to farrow their young. The veterinarian gave up on them, and they were scheduled for slaughter. Young Owen, however, elected to absent himself from school for three weeks; he delivered three hundred piglets, saving the herd. Because of this experience, Owen elected to become a veterinarian. His father, however, persuaded him to set his future sights on human medicine instead. During one summer on the farm, Owen's primary task was hauling manure, prompting him in later years to describe his quest in medicine as an aspiration "through portals of pigs and manure."

After obtaining a BA degree from the University of Minnesota, Owen entered medical school at the University of Minnesota, graduating in 1922, first in his class. Initially, he was attracted to internal medicine, but the lectures of Dr. Arthur Strachauer, the chief of the Department of Surgery at Minnesota, convinced him that surgery was "where the action was." He interned at Minnesota, but because there was no surgical residency program available at the time, he accepted a residency in medicine. Subsequently, he studied with Mayo Clinic founders Drs. William J. Mayo and Henry S. Plummer in Rochester. In 1925, he returned to the University of Minnesota to complete his PhD dissertation and examination. A possibly apocryphal story circulated implying that the examiners gave up questioning him when it was apparent that they could not find any query he could not accurately and expansively answer.

In 1929, Dr. Strachauer resigned his post as chair of surgery. A national search produced two candidates, both of whom turned down the job, one of them stating the subsequently often-quoted phrase about the school, "There is nothing here and never will be." Owen was interviewed as the third candidate and was the choice of the farsighted dean, Elias P. Lyon. Owen was only thirty-one, with the rank of instructor. The dean promoted him to assistant professor and sent him on a one-year tour of European medical institutions before making him the chair of surgery.

Owen studied with Dr. Fritz de Querain in Bern, Switzerland, and toured the German universities, becoming familiar with their broad mentorship surgery training programs. He immersed himself in extramedical culture, including reading the works of Shakespeare. Above all, he keenly observed research methodology. The European experience and his year of internal medicine convinced the young doctor that surgery could be, indeed should be, an innovative art, as well as a compendium of technical achievements in the pantheon of science.

When he returned to Minnesota, Owen was promoted to associate professor and made chair of surgery in 1930 at the age of thirty-two. In 1931, he achieved the rank of full professor. He probably was not only the youngest chair of a major department but the first to be made chairman prior to achieving the rank of full professor.

There is another apocryphal story about his early surgical practice: in the 1930s, the "downtown" private-practice surgeons exercised considerable authority over the young University of Minnesota Medical School. They attempted, allegedly, to limit Wangensteen's surgical practice to one operating room and two hospital beds. His response was to operate from early morning to nightfall, move critical patients in and out of the two beds, and lease rooms in the rowhouses that then existed across from the hospital, staffing them with nurses and hospital equipment to serve as his surgical service. In these and in other endeavors, he was supported by Dean Lyon and later Lyon's successor, Dean Harold S. Diehl. Owen Wangensteen led the way in translating laboratory research to clinical investigation. He advocated hypotheses construction, searching the known literature for prior work, taking the problem to the laboratory, and, if promising, testing the results in the clinical setting. If an innovation became standard clinical practice, he proposed ideas for improvement, and, thereby, a return to the laboratory. This circular yet progressive paradigm was the Wangensteen system.

Like Ignaz Semmelweis and Joseph Lister, pioneers in the prevention of spreading infection by the simple act of handwashing, both of whom opposed the toxin theories of their time to explain sepsis, the often fatal spread of infection to the entire body, Wangensteen rejected toxins as the primary cause of intestinal obstruction mortality, which was about 40 percent in the 1930s. He advocated for and proved that simple gaseous bowel distention, primarily from swallowed air, was the responsible agent for obstruction. For the diagnosis of bowel obstruction, he introduced auscultation of the abdomen (listening for certain bowel sounds with a stethoscope) and obtaining plain abdominal X-rays. For therapy, he prescribed intravenous fluids administration. Most important, he invented nasogastric and nasointestinal suction, later referred to as "Wangensteen suction," performed by the "Wangensteen tube." This device consisted of a rubber tube inserted through the nose, down the esophagus, to rest in the stomach or distal intestine, with the tube connected to a suction apparatus. This simple device, by evacuating intestinal gas and fluid, relieved the abdominal distention of a bowel obstruction, allowing the patient to recover spontaneously or be adequately prepared free of sepsis for interventional surgery. This innovation alone saved millions of lives and reduced the mortality of acute intestinal obstruction to below 5 percent.

Similar to the responses to Semmelweis and Lister, and to numerous medical pioneers past, present, and undoubtedly future, Wangensteen's simple and reproducible principles were at first rejected by the medical practitioners of his time. His first formal report was refused by two journals and accepted only after being repackaged under a subterfuge title. The first edition of Wangensteen's subsequent book on intestinal obstruction was originally rejected by three publishers. Surgical innovators have had to learn to persist. To those who would come under his sphere of influence, Dr. Wangensteen preached that proposing changes to accepted dogma and introducing novel therapy require, in addition to faith in one's convictions, a resilience to rejection. The ideas of the moment's majority not only can be, but often are, wrong.

Under Dr. Wangensteen's tutelage and guidance, gastrointestinal surgery flourished as a discipline. Subsequently, so did cardiovascular, transplant, and metabolic surgery. He discouraged no idea and no new direction but insisted that innovative thought be put to the test of research. In this principle of engaging in research he encouraged his faculty and his surgical trainees. He believed that exposure to a research project during residency training would provide an individual with a lifelong interest in innovation over the course of a professional career.

The diverse threads of clinical excellence, innovative thinking, research, teaching, and advocacy that constituted Owen Wangensteen's perception of surgical training would coalesce in the creation of his novel department of surgery at the University of Minnesota. His goal was to generate a department of academic surgeons training academic-minded young people to take their expertise at the University of Minnesota to other institutions, so that, in time, this country would have a cadre of surgeon-scientists. The department's unique mission would be to elevate the position of the surgeon in the United States by attainment of cognitive leadership. How well he succeeded in this aspiration was remarkable. At the end of his tenure as chairman in 1967, the graduates of his program included 38 department heads, 31 division heads, 72 directors of training programs, and 110 full professors.

The key ingredient for this enterprise was the establishment of a surgical residency with a mandatory seven-plus years, consisting of the traditional five years of clinical training supplemented by two or more years in a basic science research laboratory coincident with a return to the classroom for a PhD degree in surgery, and, whenever possible, a master's or PhD in a basic science. A surgical residency program of clinical mastery, laboratory research, and graduate scientific work was Wangensteen's unique vision. When he started this program in 1930 there was one surgical fellow in the department; by the 1950s there were up to eighty residents at any one time. Each had an individually tailored program, with faculty encouraging original thought. By 1960, about one hundred residents had graduated from the program with a PhD, including many widely recognized in surgical circles, some of them to worldwide acclaim. These included Dr. Norman Shumway, intellectual and research pioneer of heart transplantation, and Dr. Christiaan Barnard, the South African surgeon who performed the world's first heart transplant.

Wangensteen started his expansion of the residency program early in his career. In 1930, to that one surgical fellow Wangensteen added six. To obtain the requisite funds for these additions, he used the funds allocated for stipends for part-time clinical staff. The new dean, Richard E. Stammon, in a five-page letter of rebuke, reprimanded Wangensteen and threatened him with loss of his chair. Wangensteen responded in a letter in his defense: "This is a lot of trivial drivel." Dr. Wangensteen was saved in his position by the intercession of prior Dean Lyon, university president Lotus Delta Coffman, and William J. Mayo, head of the Board of Regents. Among Wangensteen's enormous accomplishments are three milestones in the discipline of surgery. In his quest to advance the progress of American surgery and to inspire young surgeons, he founded the journal *Surgery* in 1937, serving as coeditor-in-chief until 1967; this journal remains among the premier scientific venues for reporting research results. He founded the Society of University Surgeons in 1939, a professional association dedicated to showcasing the research and thoughts of young members of surgical faculties. In 1940, he originated the Surgical Forum of the American College of Surgeons. The Forum, held at the annual meeting of the American College of Surgeons, is dedicated exclusively to presentations by surgical residents and young surgeons for an audience of critical senior surgery professors. The presentations were mandated to be published as an annual bound volume.

Wangensteen was benevolent but also tough, firm, and outspoken, with little tolerance for sloth or dereliction of obligations. These traits of his were well known at Minnesota and publicly exhibited when he was president of the American Surgical Association, the oldest and most prestigious of American surgical societies. He admonished and refused the podium to a surgeon prepared to present his accepted paper because the surgeon had not complied with the requirement to hand in the paper at the time he assumed the speaker's platform. Very few people ever opposed the man known to his faculty and throughout the world of surgery as "The Chief."

Wangensteen was married twice. He had two sons and one daughter with his first wife. He lived happily with his second wife, Sarah Davidson, the first editor of the journal *Minnesota Medicine*. Sarah introduced Owen to a lifetime avocation of bird-watching to complement his pleasure in horseback riding, when his schedule allowed. He started each busy day at 4 a.m. or earlier by reading the latest and historic surgical literature.

The Minnesota legacy was originated, nourished, and sustained by Owen Wangensteen, but it is also the product, indeed the life's work, of many of his mentees, his intellectual offspring, several of whom became surgical greats. From the early roots of Wangensteen's Department of Surgery, three giants emerged who changed surgery forever. They made a worldwide impact in three major disciplines: bariatric surgery, heart surgery, and transplant surgery.

———————

Richard L. Varco was born a rancher's son in 1912 in Fairview, Montana. His early education was in a schoolhouse consisting of two to three classrooms to which he traveled on horseback. He hitched his horse to a rail with the horses of other students; when classes were over, he rode home and worked on the family ranch. When he was a young man, he wandered across the West, taking jobs at hard labor. He was relatively short, sturdy, corpulent later in life, and extremely strong. He loved to hunt and became an expert on firearms, a collector of fine rifles and shotguns. He also loved gardening, especially vegetables and flowers, cooking, and baking bread. He could have lived the life of one of the original settlers of the Great Prairie—self-reliant in nature, able to survive through physical labor, and independent in spirit.

An uncle at the University of Minnesota brought young Richard to the big city of Minneapolis to try his hand at higher education. He raced through the college and medical school curricula, obtaining his MD in 1937. In addition to his formal schooling, he became a voracious reader of nonfiction, primarily of histories, biographies, and the writings of great men. His life's hero, who he quoted liberally, was Albert Einstein. He had no patience with the make-believe world of novels and stated that the nuances of poetry totally escaped him.

After finishing medical school, Varco was at a loss to decide which field he would enter. He tried a year or so in radiology and psychiatry before he fell under the sway of Wangensteen and became his brilliant, full-time fellow. He voiced his disinclination for other fellows to join the program, stating that there was not enough surgery to go around. Wangensteen replied that he would not only increase the volume of surgery but would provide the time necessary for fellows to engage in basic laboratory research. After Varco obtained his PhD in surgery in 1940, he joined the faculty at Minnesota and became a full professor in 1950.

Wangensteen learned the technical aspects of surgery from the surgeons of his day in Minnesota and abroad, and he became an above-average craftsman, capable of performing the extended extirpative cancer surgery of the mid-twentieth century. Varco, on the other hand, not only learned by watching but was a *natural,* a virtuoso by a gift of nature. His operative basics of cutting, dissecting, separating tissues, knot tying, and sewing, all with either hand, made him capable of operating on any organ in any part of the body, for any purpose. He had huge hands, yet was ever so delicate in his touch, so that it was he who was requested to perform intricate surgery on children, even newborns.

In addition to his original ideas and surgical innovations, Varco was the surgeon who other surgeons at Minnesota consulted on how to develop, reflect upon, and improve their concepts. When a new procedure was ready for the operating room, Varco was asked to scrub in and guide the surgery. In 1952, he guided F. John Lewis and C. Walton Lillehei in performing the first open-heart operation in the world. Within ten minutes, under hypothermic cardiac arrest in which the patient's temperature was radically lowered, they repaired an atrial septal defect, a hole in the upper chambers of the heart, in a five-year old girl who subsequently lived and flourished. In 1953, Varco performed the first intestinal bypass operation specifically to incite massive weight loss for the management of obesity. For decades, he was not credited as the originator of bariatric (obesity) surgery, because he never published this lone case.

In 1954, Varco was instrumental in designing and performing the first open-heart operation using cross-circulation of blood from a father to his child, using the adult as a human heart-lung machine. This procedure was the predecessor of the invention of the bubble pump oxygenator, the mainstay of open-heart surgery, created by Richard DeWall, another talent who was given opportunity and laboratory support at Minnesota by Wangensteen.

Varco totally shunned the limelight, leaving recognition and accolades for others. He refused to speak to the media; he declined to have a facility, a laboratory, an amphitheater, or conference room named after him. He reluctantly accepted the Albert Lasker Clinical Medical Research Award in 1955. He rejected the use of the substantial money he contributed to the University of Minnesota to fund a Varco chair in surgery. He did not aspire to be a department head and turned down several such opportunities, including one at Columbia University.

Varco was a gruff man. Most residents and staff feared his uncompromising criticism and his often caustic, alarmingly candid reprimands given on his clinical service, at departmental grand rounds, and complication conferences, as well as at national surgical meetings. He did not tolerate fools. He was not a believer in support groups or life coaches for aspiring surgeons. He never complimented anyone, because he believed that being allowed the privilege of becoming a surgeon was the ultimate reward and required no words of praise. The position itself, to him, was honor achieved.

To his patients, however, Varco was kind, caring, available, even gentle. He took their problems most seriously and spent countless hours thinking about how he could make their lives better—indeed, often how to save their lives and restore them to health. He was deferential to those he respected outside of surgery. And to women he was always courteous and respectful, a true gentleman. In his private life, he shared a long and happy marriage with Louise, with whom he had eight children who not only held him in great esteem but adored him as well.

———

Clarence Walton Lillehei, formally known as C. Walton Lillehei and informally as Walt, was to become known as the father of Open-Heart Surgery. He was one of three sons of Clarence and Elizabeth Lillehei of Minneapolis. His father was a dentist; one of his brothers, Richard, became a noted University of Minnesota surgeon, and the other, James, became an esteemed internist and cardiologist in the Minneapolis–St. Paul community. Born in 1918, Walt Lillehei served with distinction in World War II on the Italian front and was awarded the Bronze Star for Valor. He achieved four degrees at the University of Minnesota: BS, MD, MS in physiology, and PhD in surgery. In 1951, he joined the Wangensteen faculty and declared his fascination with the nascent field of cardiovascular surgery. He was encouraged in this endeavor by "The Chief" and often vilified by the medical faculty for what they considered an adventurous undertaking. The early derision by some of his medical peers did not deter Lillehei. He was impervious to adverse criticism.

After considerable laboratory experimentation, Lillehei decided that he was ready to attempt an open-heart operation. On September 2, 1952, he participated in the world's first successful open-heart operation. On March 24, 1954, he converted his operative approach from hypothermia to cross-circulation to repair a ventricular septal defect, an early fatal affliction at that time. That operation was not successful, and the thirteen-month-old child died. In the face of attempts to shut down his cardiac program, Lillehei persisted. Supported by Wangensteen, he went on to perform forty-four more open-heart procedures under cross-circulation, thirty-two of which were successful in infants who would otherwise have suffered an early death.

By 1955, together with Richard DeWall, Lillehei developed the bubble pump oxygenator that circulated the patient's blood through a container in which oxygen was bubbled into the blood and carbon dioxide removed; this heart-lung machine allowed the patient's lungs to be collapsed and the heart to be arrested for surgery. With this tool, modern open-heart surgery was launched. Lillehei went on to tackle far more difficult congenital heart defects. He planned and executed repairs for children with atrial ventricular canal defects and the tetralogy of Fallot, congenital incapacitating abnormalities that, until then, resulted in limited patient survival.

Together with Earl Bakken, the founder of Medtronic, Lillehei developed the external, and then the implantable, cardiac pacemaker. He designed several cardiac valve prostheses. He was among the first, working with two Israeli surgeons, Drs. Moshe Gueron and Morris Levy, to perform and demonstrate the utility of cardiac catheterization.

Wangensteen granted Lillehei an independent cardiovascular surgery service, designated as Green Surgery. Postresidency fellows, as well as more senior surgeons, came to him for mentorship; his was probably the first cardiac surgery fellowship in the world. He trained more than 150 cardiac surgeons from more than forty countries.

Lillehei received much-deserved recognition in his lifetime, including the Albert Lasker Award in 1955, together with his mentor, Dr. Richard Varco, and with Dr. Morley Cohen and Dr. Herbert Warden.

Lillehei married Katherine (Kaye) Lindberg. They had three sons, two of whom became physicians, and one daughter. Kaye was a dynamic force in her own right, the focal point of their family life. During Lillehei's time in training an episode occurred that may have been instrumental in shaping his determination. To save his own life, he chose to risk it by undergoing a singular operative approach, never previously performed and probably never repeated. For several weeks, he had noticed large lymph nodes in his left neck that persisted and grew. A biopsy revealed a malignant lymphoma. At the time, there was no chemotherapy for this disease, a systemic cancer of the body's lymph nodes. Wangensteen reasoned that if there were no lymph nodes to become afflicted, a cure might be achieved. Thus, on one long day in the operating room, three surgeons—Wangensteen, Varco, and Arnold Kremen—removed Lillehei's lymph nodes from both sides of his neck, from under his arms, from his groins, and from his entire chest and abdominal cavities, opening his body from top to bottom. Lillehei survived, and the cancer did not. Subsequent photographs and portraits of him show his head leaning to his left, as if he had no neck muscles on that side. Indeed, he had none, because the major cervical muscle, the sternocleidomastoid, had been resected.

———

Richard Carlton Lillehei, born in 1927, formally known as Richard C. Lillehei and informally as Rich, was the younger brother of Walt. His education, including college and medical school, where he was first in his class, was at the University of Minnesota, except for two years at the Walter Reed Army Institute of Research in Bethesda, Maryland. He received his PhD in surgery in 1960 and joined the Wangensteen faculty.

Rich Lillehei was pugnacious, striving to emerge from the shadow of both his older brother Walt and Varco. Indeed, he worked extremely hard to outdo them both. At the same time, this most independent spirit was a superb mentor for the resident staff. He was aware of when they were faltering or about to make a foolish personal decision, and unobtrusively drew them aside for wise counseling. His caring nature was evident when it came to his family, especially his social, highly competent, and energetic wife, BJ (Elizabeth Jeanne) Larsen, and their four sons, two of whom became doctors.

In his abbreviated lifetime, Rich Lillehei was an excellent general and heart surgeon. He was an early transplant surgeon and, after performing multiple kidney transplants, was the first, in 1966, to transplant a pancreas; he was also a pioneer of intestinal, both small and large bowel, transplantation, one of the few surgeons ever to attempt this feat. He invented methods for organ preservation for portage between institutions, thereby greatly increasing the volume of feasible donor organs. He was one of the first to organize surgical intensive care units, and he contributed to the knowledge of patient resuscitation from posttraumatic shock.

———

The tenor of an institution is the product of its founders and their successors. What made the Minnesota program unique? What gave the Minnesota program its perspective beyond the individual characteristics of its faculty and resident body? Why did this unusual program arise when and where it did? The answer to these questions may be geographic.

The eastern medical schools were rigid in discipline, priding themselves on a European code of conduct. The manner of dress was the same throughout the East Coast: house staff uniforms of white trousers, a white shirt, a conservative tie, white shoes, and a short white jacket. The faculty, referred to as "attendings," wore conservative dress under a long white coat. For patient rounds, the service team gathered and waited for the arrival of the attending. For conferences, the students, residents, and faculty stood when the chair entered the room. No house staff ever addressed an attending on a first-name basis. On the open ward, the charity surgery services, the named procedures (e.g., appendectomy) were assigned to interns or residents depending on their years in training, which, rather than individual skills, dictated progress from simple to more complex operations. The path from intern to junior to senior to chief resident in the training program was pyramidal. After five years, only a single resident was head chief resident, the lone survivor of a class of twelve interns. The discards of these elite programs had to find lesser residencies or change their vocational plans.

This all-pervading chain of command structure extended to expressions of thought and action. The opinion of the intern was rarely requested; the dictates of the attendings were not questioned; and authority ascended with faculty rank, so that full professors—certainly not the chair—were never contradicted. Grand rounds did not consist of an exchange of ideas and, perhaps, new perspectives, but instead were scheduled affairs with formal lectures by staff, who were never disputed, on predetermined topics. The young worked to rise through these ranks, their goal being to reach the top and themselves become infallible. Too often, the result was not only a lack of progress but a perpetuation of traditions that might result not only in bad teaching, but poor patient care.

To be fair, it should be stated that in the more elite East Coast educational institutions of the past, many of the attendings worked extremely hard and kept long hours. A substantial number of them were independently wealthy, did not require a paycheck, and were driven to work in their personal limousines. They worked out of a sense of noblesse oblige, sublimating their personal ambitions to offer outstanding patient care. This cadre, as well as other highly motivated individuals, was the saving grace of the East Coast medical system.

Wangensteen, Varco, the Lilleheis, and others in the Minnesota system were Midwesterners or Westerners. They grew up with backgrounds and attitudes often grounded in some kind of physical labor, working the land. Their surroundings were not crowded; self-reliance was taken for granted. Respect for parents and elders was part of the culture, but respect for authority was not. Above all, innovation was necessary to success. Freedom of thought and expression were as wide open as the prairie.

This freedom of thought and expression was the spirit of the Wangensteen Department of Surgery. There was no dress code: residents dressed cleanly and modestly. Although shirts and ties were fairly obligatory, there were no white shoes, white trousers, or white jackets. House staff and attendings both wore long white coats. Attendings could elect to wear business suits. On the surgery services, almost everyone wore only scrubs. There was no pecking order as to who had to arrive first for rounds or conferences. All patients were treated equally, whether self-paying, covered by private insurance, or supported by the state. There were no twelve- to sixteen-bed open wards. Patients occupied single-, two-, and four-bed rooms. Each patient, regardless of financial status, was under the care of an attending and the service of that attending's house staff. No service was relegated to being a house staff ward with no or minimal supervision. Technical surgical responsibility was not regimented but dictated by natural skills, hard work, earned trust, experience, and the judgment of the attending surgeon. The pyramid residency was abolished in favor of filling the lower ranks with residents who had preselected a career in a surgical specialty, such as orthopedics. Above all, everyone was free to offer an opinion. Dialogue could become confrontational, and discussions were open to new ideas. All believed that it was the job, the privilege, actually the mandate, of the program to move beyond the status quo.

In perspective, it may be appropriate to state that emancipation from eastern medicine came from the American Midwest.

✳ 3 ✳

Settling into Minnesota

Things change, anti-Semitism remains.

ELIE WIESEL, address at Cooper
Union, November 19, 2014

On arriving in Minneapolis that September in 1960, we checked into the Curtis Hotel, an inexpensive residency hotel at the edge of downtown Minneapolis. In later years, this facility was purchased by the municipal authorities and transformed into a half-way house. Our accommodations were simple: one room with a double bed and a crib for Jane, a bathroom, and a kitchenette. After a lifetime of living in city apartments and in a Wherry housing unit at Offutt Air Force Base, we wanted a house, our first house ever, for a home.

The next morning, I reported to Dr. Wangensteen. He seemed genuinely pleased to see me, and, with a wink, stated that his letter to General Power apparently had no influence on my discharge date from the Air Force. He was referring to a letter he had sent to the four-star SAC commanding officer stating that the training program at Minnesota started on July 1, and that I should, therefore, be discharged two and a half months before my two-year service commitment ended. I don't know if General Power ever replied, but on greeting me one day, he asked me who this Wangensteen thought

34

he was, and said that, of course, I would not receive an early discharge.

Dr. Wangensteen assigned me to start on White Surgery the next day. There were six surgical services at Minnesota, each designated by a color. White, Red, and Blue were general surgery services, each staffed with more than one member of the faculty; Green, Orange, and Purple were the exclusive domains of Walt Lillehei, Richard Varco, and "The Chief," for whom the color of royalty was reserved.

Throughout our brief interview, his office door was open and our conversation was heard by Mrs. Hans, his personal secretary, who made it her business to know most departmental affairs and to influence Dr. Wangensteen's decisions when she found it necessary to do so. She came into the office, saying, "Dr. Wangensteen, he has just arrived with his wife and a child. They have as yet no permanent place to live. He cannot start work tomorrow." Dr. Wangensteen, who rarely thought of practical realities, immediately recanted his instructions for my start date and told me to take a week, or as long as I needed. I thanked him, and on my way out I thanked Mrs. Hans. I had just reached the fourth-floor elevators in the Mayo building when I heard running footsteps. Dr. Wangensteen signaled to me that I should wait and reached into his pocket for his wallet, saying he could not pay me until I actually started but that he wished to give me some money to tide me over. I refused his gracious offer and told him that we were not financially needy because we had saved all my Air Force hazardous duty flight pay.

The next day, we began looking for a house. Because we had never owned a house, or even lived in one, we were ignorant about the process of purchasing one. We contacted a realty firm and were shown available homes in our price range within a twenty- to thirty-minute drive from the University Hospital. We found to our pleasure that there were a number of desirable residential areas in

Minneapolis as well as in the adjacent suburbs or incorporated cities. One such area was the Kenwood district, located within a few blocks of Lake Calhoun (now Bde Maka Ska), Lake of the Isles, and Cedar Lake, three of the four lakes within South Minneapolis. We found a two-story wood-frame house in this location that we liked. Before committing ourselves, however, we had the good sense to hire an independent appraiser, who informed us that the plumbing and the electrical wiring were faulty and that the inner wall space might be showing some rot. In essence, the house would, he said, "nickel-and-dime" us to death. This revelation taught us how ill prepared we were to buy a house, especially in a week's time. We abandoned the idea of purchasing a home and pursued house rental advertisements. We decided that choosing the best school district would be our primary objective. Several people told us that the best schools were in the city of Edina, a suburb south of Minneapolis.

What we did not know, and what we did not find out for at least five more years, was that in the 1950s Minneapolis was known as the anti-Semitic capital of the United States. The Jews who lived in Minneapolis resided, for the most part, in St. Louis Park. At that time, there were no Jews in Edina. Totally unaware of any prejudice, and without difficulty, we rented a house in Edina and called it home for nine years. We did not have knowledge of the anti-Semitic history of our neighborhood until some years later when Jewish friends told us that, most assuredly, we were the first Jews to live in Edina.

As children of the Holocaust, we lived through an era during which mass hatred and pogroms had descended into genocide. Although we felt safe in our adopted country, we knew that certain companies, banks, and other establishments did not hire Jews. We were aware of public billboards advertising new residential opportunities in the suburbs of New York City that openly stated in large letters "Restricted," meaning "no Jews." We knew that our colleges, as well as my medical school, probably had a Jewish quota. I have already described the anti-Semitism pervasive in surgical residency programs in the East.

There was certainly no anti-Semitism in the Department of Surgery at Minnesota. The only prejudice Dr. Wangensteen exhibited was against people who failed to work hard and make the most of their potential. The story is told that early in his career "The Chief" became aware that there were excellent surgeons and a splendid research program at the Mt. Sinai Hospital. This facility was established by the philanthropic generosity of Jay Phillips, one of the largest liquor dealers in the Midwest, who wanted a clinical facility for Jewish physicians because they were routinely barred from the better private hospitals and from the University. Dr. Wangensteen befriended Mr. Phillips, and they developed a kinship based on their common striving for excellence. Dr. Wangensteen appointed a Department of Surgery faculty member to oversee a newly established university Department of Surgery residency rotation at Mt. Sinai. Jewish doctors were not only welcomed into the Wangensteen residency but Dr. Wangensteen brought them onto his faculty. These ecumenical initiatives circumvented the various religious and ethnic prejudices of Minneapolis and St. Paul, and effectively destroyed flagrant anti-Semitism in the medical community of the Twin Cities. In 1976, a thirteen-story clinical and office building of the University of Minnesota Medical School was erected on campus and named the Phillips-Wangensteen Building.

We were fortunate to find a rental house with a detached garage in Edina within a twenty-minute drive of downtown Minneapolis and the university. Minnehaha Creek ran along one side of our rental house, within three feet of its slab foundation. Across the creek was heavily wooded, hilly municipal land. This tucked-away alcove had no traffic. Children could play on the little lawn at the side of the house, and in the sandbox and on the tire swing I built.

To one side of the house was a small grassy area with a single-unit redwood picnic table and bench seats. Walking along the creek, one reached a park with a large lawn, also furnished with play equipment. On the far side of the park was a hill perfect for winter sledding. In the summer, when the creek was high, many people, including our family, rubber-tubed down the creek. In the winter, the creek was a pleasant venue for skating.

The front door to our redwood house was on the north side through a small screened porch. From the start, we rarely used this entrance, and soon it became the space for our dog's insulated dog-house. The extremely brief entryway from the front door flowed to the right into the living/dining area, which ran the length of the house on the creek side. Immediately in front of the entry was the staircase to the upper story; to the left, a bathroom and a room we furnished as a playroom. On the west side of the stairs was the side entrance, the one we and our guests regularly used leading through the furnace room and laundry. On the south side of the first floor was our small kitchen and dinette area. Our bedroom was at the top of the stairs to the right, and to the left a cubicle of a room, advertised as a "sewing room," as well as a half-bath and the hall-way to the children's bedroom. Our furnishings were simple. The long living room on the main floor held brick-and-wood book-cases we built; other highlights included a mahogany and marble coffee table I made in my spare time in the workshop at Offutt as well as the high-fidelity speakers I assembled from separate sound and player components housed in wooden cabinets I made. A gui-tar rack for Daisy, who played and sang the folk songs of the fifties and sixties completed my woodworking efforts, which I stopped for lack of time and out of concern for the safety of my fingers.

Our house was owned by George Speakes, the proprietor of the American Rug Laundry. His father lived in the small white house at the south end of the turnaround. He was cantankerous, reclusive, and surly when he emerged from his home. I made an effort to befriend him, and he invited us into his house. As he became more loquacious, he started to pour out his anti-Semitic convictions. We subsequently limited our interactions to leaving our monthly rental check for his son with him. George Speakes had a young daughter he doted on and to whom he had willed our house. On several occasions, he refused to sell us the house and property, which we hoped to purchase and expand. George was extremely fond of this small jewel of a residence and cherished the thought of his daughter, in her maturity, residing there. Several years after we moved away, George died. When his daughter inherited the house, she promptly sold it.

The Andersons were our neighbors and became good friends. Ron was an engineer and Bev, his soulmate. She and Daisy traded foods and recipes. Their three children were friends with ours. The children were brought up strictly, with good manners. David, the youngest, was often in trouble but was a sweet child who always addressed me as "Mr. Dr. Buchwald." A memorable moment with the Andersons came during a tornado warning. I was at the hospital, and Bev brought Daisy, the kids, and our German shepherd dog Buck over to their house to shelter in their basement huddled together during the storm.

Midway down the dirt road lived the Josephsons. Mr. Josephson and I traded stories. He was a World War II veteran, a marine who had seen considerable combat island-hopping in the Pacific. He promised himself that if he survived he would barbecue a steak on an outdoor grill every evening of his life. This he did, for at least as long as we lived there. Summer or winter, on my way home, I would wave to him as he grilled. When we shared drinks, I would often lecture him on the evils of cholesterol and eating red meat as his steaks were cooking. He would simply laugh at my warnings, saying that after what he had gone through, he was living on borrowed time anyway.

Before we left Offutt, Daisy was offered a position as a teaching assistant and PhD graduate student in the Department of English at the University of Minnesota. We interviewed several candidates as part-time babysitters for our daughter. One said she loved to drive and would drive Jane around the Twin Cities each day. She was not hired. We employed two others for a brief time. Then along came Mamie—Mary Boruski—who soon became a member of our family. Her husband, Ray, had survived combat in World War II only to die of a heart attack in 1945. Mamie never remarried and had no children. She was extremely close to her sister and her family. She was with us for about ten years, taking superlative part-time care of our growing family. She was a disciplinarian with our children and our giant German shepherd dog. She was caring, intelligent, protective, and loving. Mamie was a devout Catholic, a member of the Third Order of Dominicans. She performed extraordinary church duties and was granted the privilege of being buried in the habit of a Dominican nun. I helped in her terminal care but could do little else except visit and hold her hand. She was buried in the Fort Snelling National Cemetery, next to her husband, who she always referred to as "my darling boy."

Parking was difficult at the university. Daisy generally took the bus to and from work, changing buses in all weather conditions. She taught Freshman English for a few years, and then courses in Shakespeare studies. Her PhD adviser was the celebrated eighteenth-century scholar Samuel Monk.

My first day of work as a junior resident was eventful. I was assigned to White Surgery, the service of Dr. J. (Joseph) Bradley Aust, and I was on my way to scrub with him when I ran into Jack

Bloch, from my intern days at P&S. He had started his residency at Minnesota on leaving the National Institutes of Health (NIH) that past June. To find a best friend unexpectedly was an amazing discovery, and it offered the happy prospect of many years of working together. We talked for only a few minutes that day and made a date for Daisy and me to meet Gretchen, a nurse he married while at the NIH, and their newborn son, Rob.

My first operation in Minnesota was a hemicorporectomy, that is, removal of the lower half of the body. An unfortunate paraplegic had developed a widely spreading perineal cancer, and a local resection would have been fruitless. Joe Aust reasoned that, because the man had no use of his legs or normal stool and bladder function, he could remove the entire malignancy by cutting the man's body in half, closing the torso with a healthy flap of muscle, fat, and skin, providing the patient with a colostomy and a urinary conduit. Indeed, more of the patient went to pathology than remained in the operating room. The operation took the entire day. The patient recovered and left the hospital with a special motorized chair and a trapeze apparatus for his bed. When Daisy asked me what I had done on my first day in the operating room, I responded, "You don't want to know."

The 1950s and 1960s in American surgery were the heyday of massive, radical cancer resections. With the advent of reliable anesthesia allowing for the safe prolongation of surgery and the availability of better instrumentation, and considering the meager nonsurgical options of the time, surgeons pursued a no-limits approach to resectability. This concept was based on the belief that removal of the primary malignancy and contiguous tissues could, in many circumstances, elicit a cure. Indeed, it was the only hope for a cancer cure at that time.

In accord with this concept, the radical mastectomy for cancer of the breast was extended from encompassing the axillary lymph nodes to the mediastinal and supraclavicular lymph nodes, and even the underlying muscle and ribs of the chest wall. Disfiguring facial and neck operations, with removal of the larynx and thus the ability for normal speech, were also widely practiced. Another procedure that was introduced during that time was pelvic exenteration for carcinoma of the endometrium of the uterus. This operation involved not only removal of the uterus and ovaries, but the rectum and bladder as well, with construction of colonic and bladder ostomies. In retrospect, this era of surgical technical heroics sometimes cured, often palliated, and frequently extended life expectancy for some, but at a significant cost.

My first night on call was essentially sleepless, with a continuous stream of patient problems and emergencies to attend to. Nonetheless, I was happy and it felt good getting back to surgical life. I was in fine spirits, watching the sun rise at 6 a.m. I had not had time for breakfast before morning rounds and the operating room at 7 a.m. I went to the refrigerator on the nursing station and removed a small orange-juice container sealed with a plastic top. As I was drinking the juice, I was confronted by the hospital director who informed me who he was. I was later to learn that there was a fictitious award in his name for penny-pinching. The director told me that I was stealing juice designated for patients. He took my name and said he would report me to Dr. Wangensteen and to the dean. I elected not to respond, neither offering an explanation nor telling him where he could go. I walked away from a confrontation. That afternoon, I was paged by Dr. Wangensteen. I heard the laughter in his voice when he said, "So, we have an orange-juice thief in our midst." He went on: "You have now been spoken to. If the dean's office calls you, tell them to call me. I'll take care of this, Dr. Buchwald. You have, I believe, more important uses for your time." One more chuckle from Dr. Wangensteen and he was off the line. He required no explanation from me. He had been a surgical resident; he was a surgeon; he was raising the next generation of surgeons. I am certain that during many a night, or early in the morning, he had "stolen" many an orange juice from the station refrigerator.

✤ 4 ✤

Culture Shock

*It must be heartening to
undergraduate medical students to see
how fallible their professors are.*

OWEN H. WANGENSTEEN, *New England
Journal of Medicine*, 1952

My surgical childhood at P&S of Columbia University was permeated by the stultified East Coast tradition I have already described. I was accustomed to a dress code, an overstated insistence on deference, a chain-of-command structure that established the veracity of knowledge, and, above all, social and communication barriers based on seniority, rank, and background. In our initial brief conversation on my arrival in Minnesota, my friend Jack Bloch told me to expect an entirely different culture. I was, however, not prepared for the actual experience of becoming part of the Minnesota Department of Surgery system of personal interactions, informality of dress and address, and total absence of obsequiousness. At Minnesota, ascendency in responsibility, rank, or respect was not based on the passage of time or on an unspoken command to avoid controversy. Each man (at the time, there were no women in academic surgery) was expected to be an individual who determined his own success or failure.

On my first day on White Surgery, Professor Joe Aust, head of the service, insisted that I address him as Joe or Brad. On day two of my residency, I went to his outpatient clinic. He had given me strict instructions about a specific patient. I carried them out. Then a resident appeared who totally countermanded Dr. Aust's orders, even when I told him that these were Dr. Aust's wishes. He informed me that he was Dr. Aust's associate and that I was to do only as he said. Further, he told me that I should address him as doctor, not by his first name. When Dr. Aust came to clinic, he was irate and demanded to know why I had not carried out his orders. I replied, "Joe, your associate, told me not to and gave me new orders." He responded: "That man is the third-year resident in my laboratory. He is a resident just like you. I am the professor of surgery in charge of White Surgery." Thus, in addition to a certain atmosphere of informality, there were several unusual individuals present and tolerated in the program. I was the victim of a prankster or an eccentric. Either way, the resident's unusual behavior that day, and on other occasions, was ignored by the faculty because he was clever and he was performing original work in the laboratory.

Another example of tolerance for quirky behavior involved a fellow on Dr. Walt Lillehei's Green Surgery service. This man, a visiting surgery fellow from Turkey called the local press on his own responsibility and asked them to be present for Tuesday's afternoon Mortality and Morbidity Conference for a special, extraordinary scientific announcement. Toward the end of the conference, the room suddenly filled with reporters. The fellow rose, embraced Dr. Wangensteen, and exclaimed, "In the glorious reign of Dr. Owen H. Wangensteen, in the era of Dr. C. Walter Lillehei, I have discovered an agent that will lyse clots and, thereby, put an end to clotted arteries and veins forever." He went on speaking; the reporters made notes and asked questions. Dr. Wangensteen inched toward the door, calling for Dr. Aust to free him from this unwelcome confrontation. Dr. Wangensteen kept repeating, "Oh my! oh my!"—his favorite exclamation when surprised by an adverse event. The story ran in the local papers. The "great discovery," however, turned out to be an anticoagulant commonly placed into test tubes to prevent blood used for analysis from clotting. Given intravenously, the anticoagulant would be toxic and probably fatal. Dr. Walt Lillehei, who did not attend the conference, dismissed the incident as humorous. That was the end of it. The fellow finished his scheduled Minnesota tenure and returned to Turkey.

At the time of my arrival in Minnesota in 1960, the Green Surgery service was the only postresidency specialty service. This service was dedicated to heart surgery and existed as an independent entity, solely under the direction of Dr. Walt Lillehei. All the other services were general surgery services, encompassing a common residency program, with assignment to a specific service at the direction of Dr. Wangensteen and Dr. Aust, presumably after consultation with the head of that particular unit. As stated earlier, Dr. Richard L. Varco was in charge of Orange Surgery and Dr. J. Bradley Aust headed White Surgery.

Dr. John F. Perry, a Texan, was the chief of Blue Surgery. He was an excellent surgeon and teacher, well liked by all and a favorite of the residents. A true generalist in his practice, he was skilled in all phases of surgical practice and specialized in none. John had a difficulty unusual in a surgeon—a gross tremor of his hands, a tremor that, as if by magic, totally ceased when he picked up a surgical instrument.

Dr. Richard Lillehei was at the time the junior attending on Red Surgery, which was under the supervision of Dr. Alan Thal, a mercurial personality, highly intelligent, with broad research interests.

Thal was interested in me. Somehow, he had found out that as a medical student I had constructed a sensitive, microassay apparatus to measure serum histamine. The apparatus was not commercially available; its prototype and only other embodiment was at

Columbia University P&S where I built it. Why Thal wanted this apparatus he never divulged to me. Jack Bloch and several faculty members told me to be wary of him. I also heard this amusing anecdote about Thal: A resident by the name of Rosenkrantz called Thal about a patient one evening. Knowing that Thal started life as Rosenthal, he opened the conversation by saying, "Hello, Thal. This is Krantz." In my first month in Minnesota, I spent off-duty hours building the histamine apparatus in Thal's laboratory but politely refused his offer to come into his laboratory later in my residency training.

In addition to Joe Aust, White Surgery was staffed by two other surgeons: Dr. Theodor Grage and Dr. W. Albert Sullivan. Although I joined the residency only during the last month of the four-month summer rotation, I was nevertheless accepted in Minnesota fashion by the White Surgery faculty: there was no inequality based on academic rank or age, a familiarity unthinkable back east. This was yet another culture shock for me.

Al Sullivan immediately befriended me, as he had done so many times with others in his role as dean of students and surgery mentor; he made me feel as if we shared a common background, which we did not. He was a southern gentleman, educated at Tulane, who spent considerable time practicing medicine in Paris, becoming fluent in the French language before coming to the University of Minnesota. His tenure in France was interrupted by service in a MASH unit in Korea. He was known for his fairness, decency, and gentleness, in and out of the operating room—a man whose character was completely the opposite of the general perception of the rough-and-ready surgical personality. He was by far the best didactic teacher and instructor in operating-room principles and etiquette in the department.

Sullivan also had a wry sense of humor and was quick-witted in his responses. I recall an occasion when we were having lunch

together in the hospital cafeteria. This facility periodically changed
its rules for meal selection. At one time, the rule was that you could
have as much of any item as you wished but that you could not
have any other item with it. For breakfast, this edict separated eggs
from bacon. Thus, when Jack Bloch and I breakfasted together, I
would order four sunny-side up eggs and Jack two orders of bacon.
We would then sit down and divide our dishes. One morning, the
matron in charge of the cafeteria came over and took our plates
away, saying to Jack, "You can't eat his eggs," and to me, "You can't
eat his bacon." The same person was behind the service counter
when Al and I came through on another day. The cafeteria rules,
however, had changed; now you could have different items in your
dish selection, but you could no longer take more than one portion
of a particular dish. Al, for unfathomable reasons, liked the cafeteria's chocolate pudding and placed two servings of it on his tray.
The cafeteria dictator came charging over and yelled at him, "You
can't have two chocolate puddings." Al instantly took a third, "I'm
sorry; I'll take three." The woman was rendered speechless, and we
moved on.

My relationship with Theodor (Ted) Grage was excellent from
the start. In his teens, Ted had manned an antiaircraft gun in Nazi
Germany. After World War II, he completed his basic education
in Germany and then moved to the United States, where he finished medical school in Omaha before coming to the University of
Minnesota. He married an American, Mary Ann Parks, a vivacious
freethinker who was a willing tap-dance performer at parties. The
Grages had seven children and were a tight family unit. In addition
to being a hunter, Ted was an avid gardener, raising a huge selection
of vegetables, including kohlrabi, little known in the United States.

Ted hated totalitarianism, Hitler, and Nazism. Unlike some
Germans I have met who speak as if the Nazis and Hitler had
descended from outer space and simply disappeared from the Earth

after the war, he acknowledged and abhorred the crimes of his fellow citizens. His remorse and empathy for the murdered and displaced generations of millions of Jews was genuine. Although he loved things German, made his own sausages, quoted Goethe, and epitomized the no-nonsense German autocrat, he detested those who assumed an intrinsic conviction of superiority and an insistence on dominance. He was gregarious. He was the first member of the faculty to build a backyard swimming pool for his children, where he entertained their friends and his. In the summer, the Grages threw huge informal parties with hearty food and a great variety of alcoholic beverages. On leaving White Surgery at the end of October 1960, Daisy and I attended our first of several parties at the Grages. We had a grand time and felt ever so welcomed into the Minnesota Department of Surgery family.

Joe Aust was an avid tennis player. When he found out that I played tennis, he immediately invited me to play with him. For the next several years, we played tennis together almost every Sunday, weather permitting, at a public cement court close to his home. Joe played with ferocity and always to win. I was a decent-enough player, and we were fairly evenly matched. After a morning on the courts, Joe and I often would go to his house to have brunch with his pleasant wife, Connie.

This surprising and unexpected receptiveness of faculty toward residents was startling but paled in comparison to the culture shock I experienced at my first Saturday grand rounds.

Grand rounds was a tradition in almost all teaching medical centers, and in many community and private hospitals. At the elite East Coast academic establishments, grand rounds were fairly formulaic: The surgery staff, fellows, and residents gathered for two to three hours on a designated day and time in an amphitheater. A patient was rolled in on a gurney. The patient looked about at the audience, possibly amused or frightened, and almost certainly perplexed. A resident talked about the patient, presenting his or her problem, evaluation, and therapy, past and planned. At times, staff would descend into the pit of the amphitheater and talk to or examine the patient. After the resident's presentation, the patient was rolled out. A planned and probably rehearsed discourse by a previously designated member of the attending staff followed. There was no discussion and certainly no disputing commentary. The next patient was rolled in and the performance was repeated. Two to three such semididactic presentations were usually followed by a lecture from a visiting professor or a member of the faculty. When this talk was completed and perfunctory praise had been offered and benign questions answered, grand rounds was concluded for that week.

At Minnesota, grand rounds occurred on Saturday mornings. From 9 to II a.m. cases were discussed, and from II a.m. to noon there was a lecture. Each member of the faculty sat in a specific seat in the amphitheater, as if the seat had been assigned, or as if each occupant was a permanent ticket holder. Most of the faculty sat in the first two rows; others claimed seats farther back. A resident could sit anywhere, as long as it wasn't in a faculty chair. There is a sketch familiar to many in the hallway of the Department of Surgery showing this seating arrangement in the 1960s, with cartoon representations of the members of the faculty.

Apart from the established seating, once the conference began, all civility was abandoned. A resident presented a case, but he was frequently interrupted and questioned. A free-for-all ensued. Fortunately, rarely was a patient rolled into the room to witness the disharmony of the people responsible for his or her care. The faculty, and even occasionally the residents, argued vigorously with one other, with no holds barred. They criticized the knowledge, judgment, technical skills, competence, and at times the intelligence and personal motivation of their colleagues. This melee extended to visitors as well. In a heated argument with a visiting British surgeon who had just appealed to his years of experience, Dr. Varco, establishing his own credentials, said, "I may not be the best surgeon in the world, but I am certainly one of the best." Only Dr. Wangensteen kept above the fray, enjoying the exchanges and taking pride in the independence and powerful minds of his prodigies.

In replaying the events of my first Saturday conference to Daisy, I once again said, "You won't believe this." How lovely culture shock can be.

❧ 5 ❧

Anoka and Stillwater

Independence is happiness.

SUSAN B. ANTHONY

My first full four-month rotation started in November 1960 when I was assigned outside the University Hospital to the Anoka State Hospital and the Stillwater State Prison rotation. Anoka is about an hour's drive northwest of the university and was the primary incarceration state medical facility. Its building units housed several groups of patients: the mentally impaired; those with tuberculosis and indigent, or who refused medical therapy (a state law allowed for their incarceration); penitentiary inmates with severe, primarily pulmonary diseases; and a juvenile psychiatric unit. The Anoka surgical team during my rotation consisted of a senior fourth-year resident (Dr. Donald G. McQuarrie); a junior, second- to fourth-year resident (me); and a first-year intern. For difficult cases at Anoka, a staff member, usually Dr. Aust or Dr. Perry, would come out to assist. As the junior resident, I was also assigned to Stillwater Prison as the sole surgical representative. Stillwater Prison, the state maximum-security prison, is located southeast of Anoka and east of the university; each leg is about an hour's drive. I spent many hours driving the home/university/Anoka/Stillwater route, in addition to attending the university Saturday's grand rounds conference.

The main surgical service for nonpenitentiary patients at Anoka consisted of twelve-bed women's and men's wards, separated by a corridor and a nurses'/doctors' station. This room was accessible through a door that was paneled waist high and windowed above. I was on call and sleeping in the residents' quarters building one night, when, at about 2 a.m., I received an emergency call from the surgical unit. A female catatonic schizophrenic patient, who had not moved from her bed for months, got up and, in a crouch, crossed past the nursing station to the men's ward without being seen. Most of the men were restrained in their beds, and nearly all had Foley urinary catheters in place. Within a few minutes, she had pulled all the catheters, without deflating their retention balloons, and run back to her bed. When I arrived, there was screaming and cursing in the men's ward, with blood and urine splattered on the floor and walls, soaking the beds. I spent the rest of the night reinserting Foley catheters.

Sexual activity was alive and well at Anoka. The multiple buildings on the Anoka campus were connected by poorly lit tunnels that contained the electrical, water, and heating conduits and served as passageways for the staff, especially in the winter and at night when the various campus buildings were locked. These corridors were utilized for other purposes, particularly at night. When summoned after midnight, one was aware of couples of one sort or another in some of the alcoves coming off the main corridors. Returning one evening to the surgical residents' on-call suite of living room, bedroom, small kitchen, and bathroom, I heard sounds coming from the bedroom. I investigated and found a nude teenaged girl in my bed. I realized that she was from the juvenile psychiatric unit. I told her to dress and escorted her back to her apparently unlocked "locked" facility. Years later, one of the psychiatrists was fired for a sexual dalliance with a teenager in the unit.

We performed surgery in an ordinary room with screened windows on the second floor of one of the buildings. It was still warm in early November the year of my rotation, and the windows were partially open. Some of the screens were torn, and at times flying insects circled the operative field and were swatted away. Our superb nurse anesthetist was a middle-aged woman; she had no assistant and a weak bladder. Thus, every two hours or so, one of us had to break scrub to take over behind the ether screen to allow her to go to the bathroom. It was a different operating room climate than I was used to, but we did good work and our patients did well.

Don McQuarrie was a fine surgeon and a good teacher; he led me through several gastrectomies for ulcer disease and multiple hernia procedures. He performed the pulmonary resections with me as his first assistant. For major operations, such as an esophagectomy, attending staff would join us. I had not performed surgery as an Air Force flight surgeon, and my stint on White Surgery was for only one month. Therefore, I appreciated this opportunity to scrub routinely, see a variety of procedures, and participate in and perform surgery. Being in the operating room removed the last lingering vestige of regret about leaving the Air Force and strengthened my conviction that I was meant to be a surgeon. The operating room remained my home away from home, and so often a sanctuary that protected me, at least for a time, from the less congenial aspects of an academic career.

I not only learned how to perform different procedures but became proficient in the use of standard instruments, handling tissues delicately, obtaining adequate operative field exposure, and working as part of a surgical team. I observed my various mentors performing surgery. I admired the technique and approach of some; others failed to impress me when I found their surgery crude, wasteful of time and blood. Both extremes were teaching lessons—one provided a standard to emulate and achieve, the other to reject. I believed that I could learn to perform at the higher level of competence, and that I could and would do better than certain of the senior staff I witnessed in the operating room. Regardless of whatever reputation I might achieve as a researcher and innovator, becoming a highly competent technical surgeon, respected for my operating-room skills, was a major career goal.

On the Anoka rotation, I also refurbished my patient-care capabilities. I continuously practiced patient evaluation, diagnosis, preparation for surgery, and immediate postoperative care. I acquired facility with drug formularies and how to perform bedside procedures efficiently. I had sick patients to take care of, to understand, and to empathize with. I appreciated how fortunate I was to be a doctor on the path to becoming a surgeon.

The food at the Anoka facility was free, bland, institutional fare. For a gustatory treat, we would drive into town to the Embers franchise, long gone, for one of their charcoal-grilled hamburgers. I immensely enjoyed these outings, which remain vivid in my memory. Indeed, I can still almost taste those hamburgers and recollect the sensation of normalcy and the beauty of personal freedom that existed outside the state hospital.

———

Because Stillwater State Prison had no in-house physician, it contracted for visiting physician services, including surgical services, with the University of Minnesota Department of Surgery. Surgery needs at the prison required less than a full-time practitioner; therefore, the Department of Surgery assigned one junior resident to cover both Anoka and Stillwater prison.

This rotation was a major growth experience. I was alone. There was no one to call in for help in the operating room. I made the decisions about whether or not to perform surgery, as well as overseeing the care of the surgical patients. Above all, I did my best to obey the Hippocratic dictum "Do No Harm." In addition to my surgical education, Stillwater prison provided me with an insight into prison life and the prisoners incarcerated there. Several days a week, I held clinic hours, made rounds on the hospitalized patients, and operated. I performed many minor procedures, such as hernia repairs, and a few major operations, such as gastrectomies for ulcer disease, partial thyroidectomies, and one parotid gland excision.

The operating room at the prison was well equipped and far more modern than the one at the Anoka State Hospital. My surgical assistants were two inmates: one, with a history of violent bar robberies, was my scrub nurse; the other, a senior post-office employee who had killed his wife for infidelity, was my circulating nurse. They were both skillful and far more attentive than many an operating room nurse in the outside world. Our nurse anesthetist was a comely young woman in her thirties who came to the prison for the scheduled elective surgical procedures. After the day's surgery was completed, my two assistants would hurry me off to the hospital kitchen and close the door to the operating room suite, where they remained happily ensconced with the anesthetist for about an hour before she was escorted out of the prison.

The Stillwater hospital kitchen was under the supervision of a former airport chef serving time for embezzlement. He ran a clean establishment, very well furnished with a host of cooking implements, including, to my surprise, all sorts of knives. He prided himself on the sumptuous soufflés and omelets he made for me from simple ingredients of eggs, potatoes, onions, and herbs. He would serve these creations with a flourish, and he, the ever-present guard, and I would sit while I ate and discuss the world's problems.

The hospital ward night shift was under the care of an older inmate referred to as Nursie. He was a clever drug addict. Under the careful scrutiny of a guard, Nursie would draw up the morphine I had prescribed for my postoperative patients and return the stock bottle to the drug cabinet, the key for which was in the possession of the guard. In the presence of the guard, he would go to the patient's bedside, place the patient's arm on top of his own, and with a long needle perforate the patient's arm, enter his own arm with the needle, and give himself the narcotic. In the morning, I would find patients labeled as drug seekers and malingerers writhing in pain. Finally, Nursie was caught and replaced.

My scrub nurse was also my clinical assistant and excelled in that capacity as well. In his spare hours, he worked out in the prison gymnasium. He was most knowledgeable about muscle development, free weights, and bodybuilding. He was extremely strong. One day, a hired murderer jailed for the contract killing of a prominent person's wife came in for his usual weekly consultation for some minor problem. As the inmate was leaving, my scrub nurse caught up with him and twisted his arm behind his back. He told the prisoner that if he screamed or made any noise, he would, for starters, break his arm. I asked my scrub nurse what he was doing. He walked the inmate back to my desk and quietly said to him, "Put Doc's pen back on his desk and don't ever try to take it again." The man did as he was told. My scrub nurse gave his arm an extra twist as a warning and threw him out the door.

I soon became cognizant of the mind-set of many convicts. Although they were consistently complaining about being in prison and counting the days until their release, for some the penitentiary was their home, the environment in which they felt secure in the society of their peers, the world in which they commanded respect, and, of course, a place that provided food, shelter, medical care, minimal work, and entertainment, without the hardship of having to earn them. For many a prisoner, the loss of freedom was a small price to pay for security; freedom was more a burden than a desired privilege.

During the time of my Stillwater rotation, a man in his sixties with osteomyelitis of one of his legs, barely able to walk, served his time and was released. He returned several weeks later after being caught fleeing from the attempted robbery of a small grocery store during the day. I asked him why he had committed the crime and was so easily apprehended. He smiled conspiratorially and said, "Doc, you know how fast I can run on this leg. I pleaded guilty right away."

There is also truth to the notion that criminals tend to repeat their crimes. My scrub nurse was released several years after my tenure at the prison. I obtained a job for him as a trainer in a gymnasium. He also had a day job as a truck driver and had moved in with the anesthetist. One evening, he called me and said he had an overwhelming desire to rob a bar and start an altercation. I told him to meet me in an all-night diner. We talked until the bars closed, and I hoped that I had dissuaded him from his impulse. A few months later, I was listening to television while taking off my shoes before going to bed, and when I looked up, there was my scrub nurse on the screen. He had robbed a bar, fled into a small park, and had, of course, been apprehended.

My circulating nurse was also released and reemployed by the postal service. He came to see me one day to tell me that he had a girlfriend who was seeing someone else as well, and that he had the impulse to shoot her. I dissuaded him, stressing that he had no right to feel so possessive of a woman to whom he was not engaged, or with whom he had any other commitment. I told him that she had the right to date others, that shooting someone in a fit of passion was never justifiable, and, most certainly, that it would land him back in jail for the rest of his life. Happily, I believe he never obeyed his homicidal impulse.

My most dramatic time at Stillwater occurred one night in January. I was called at home and informed that two prisoners had been in a knife fight and that both were fairly well cut up. I drove to

Stillwater. I ascertained that there was no penetrating organ damage and repaired the superficial wounds. It was well past midnight when I was ready to leave. My first Minnesota blizzard was raging outside. The guard who led me out told me that I should not attempt to drive back to the Twin Cities but should instead stay in a spare room in the guard's quarters for the night. I declined his kind and reasonable offer. I got into my automobile, without any blankets or other emergency equipment. These were the days before cell phones. I drove off on Highway 10.

There were no other vehicles on the road. Visibility was near zero. The windshield wipers could not contend with the pelting snow. I opened the window and attempted to drive with my head out in the snowy maelstrom. I soon found the driving extremely rough. I stopped the car but had the good sense not to turn off the engine. I had driven onto a cornfield. I was a good distance from the road; corn husks were the cause of the uneven and bumpy driving surface I experienced. Somehow, I made my way back onto the highway and to a well-lit filling station. To the great surprise of the owner-attendant behind the counter, I walked in out of the storm. He told me that he lived only a mile down the road but that he was not crazy enough to have attempted to drive there. That was fortunate for me, because had he gone home I would have found the station locked. He invited me to spend the night, and I used his phone to call Daisy. He and I ate candy bars and drank soda pop from the dispensing machines. We slept on the floor until morning. By then, the storm had blown itself out, and I could, slowly and carefully, drive home. I gained great respect for blizzards.

Anoka and Stillwater were experiences I had not expected from my time in medical school and as an intern. In those settings, the patient had a disease, a malady that surgery could cure or attempt to ameliorate. The patients' intellectual capacity varied, but, if not impaired by their illness, they were mentally competent. Many had psychological problems, but they were functioning within society. If any of them were criminals, we, the house staff, were usually not aware of it. They entered of their own free will into the controlled environment of a hospital or a hospital clinic. For this four-month rotation, however, I was practicing medicine and surgery in facilities of incarceration. The patients were mentally impaired, or severely psychologically ill, dangerous to society, or exhibited elements of two or more of those conditions. Although these patients were different from those in standard community practice, they were still patients, and they were my patients.

During this rotation, I formed my lifetime credo of responsibility. If anything adverse occurred to any of my patients, I decided to believe that it was my fault; for example, if a patient fell out of bed, I should have prevented it. Some surgeons tend to blame adverse outcomes on the disease, the environment, or the patients themselves, rather than on an act, or a failure to act, of theirs. I believe that the principle of assuming ownership of the bad, as well as the good, made me a better doctor and, therefore, of greater benefit to my patients.

My medical life had changed. I was much more on my own exposed to a wide spectrum of diseases, as well as living in a medical environment very different from that of New York. I found justification for questioning certain dogma taught in my earlier years. Ridiculous as it sounds, we were taught in medical school that nervousness gave rise to hyperthyroidism rather than the reverse, that ulcers occurred in midlevel executives frustrated in their efforts to climb the corporate ladder, and that Crohn's disease of the intestine (first described at Mt. Sinai Hospital in New York) was a problem of young Jewish girls emotionally attached to their mothers. In my new surroundings, I had great difficulty envisioning my first middle-aged, phlegmatic, male, Swedish patient with Crohn's disease as a young Jewish girl. The more I learned, the more I recognized how ignorant medicine still was. The prospect of combining research with clinical surgery was an even more powerful beacon. In the Wangensteen Department of Surgery, I was in the best place to start my academic career.

✦ 6 ✦

Wangensteen's Surgery Service

All work and no play . . .

JAMES HOWELL, *Proverbs*, 1659

For my final first-year four-month rotation in 1961, I was assigned to Purple Surgery, Dr. Wangensteen's service. My fellow junior resident was Jack Bloch, the senior resident was Don McQuarrie, and our chief resident was an autocrat. With our friendship reestablished, Jack and I extended our relationship to our wives and, subsequently, to our children. Daisy and Gretchen became close friends, and the two families became an extended family. We picnicked and spent holidays and weekends together. We confided in each other, we shared triumphs as well as sorrows.

I once played a prank on Jack at work. Dr. Wangensteen had several idiosyncrasies. One was standing on a moist mat while operating, supposedly to trap bacteria. Another was having one of the residents shine the "handheld light" over his shoulder. This was a lightbulb positioned on a broomstick pole that was connected to an electric outlet because there was as yet no powerful operating room lights and headlights. One day, I was holding the "handheld light" over Dr. Wangensteen's right shoulder. I lost my concentration and my aim accidentally deviated from the operative field so

62

that the light shone instead on Dr. Wangensteen's neck. He moved
away from the hot beam. Realizing that this was an opportunity,
I periodically repeated this maneuver. Finally, Dr. Wangensteen
turned around and said, "Henry, you are too short to hold the light.
Get Dr. Bloch in here and trade places." And so I did, handing off
the "handheld light" to the six-foot-tall Jack, to whom I later con-
fessed.

Our chief resident wanted desperately to be thought of as a
great leader. He was constantly perplexed by having as his junior
residents three individuals who were more adept than he was. He
issued orders that no decision was to be made, no act to be performed, without consulting him and receiving his approval. One
day, I removed a T-tube (a T-shaped drainage catheter) from the
bile duct of a patient at the appropriate and scheduled time. My
chief resident found out and summoned me to the operating room
and shouted, "I told you to ask my advice and permission before
removing any tubes from any of my patients." I heatedly responded:
"When I want the advice of a jackass, I'll ask you." It was not politic
of me, but there were no repercussions.

On another occasion, our Purple Surgery team of four were
walking down the hall discussing a particularly grievous blunder
the chief resident had made but was not going to acknowledge. I
asked him how he would respond when Dr. Wangensteen questioned him. I had learned to mimic Dr. Wangensteen's high-pitched
voice and intonation fairly well. I placed my right forefinger and
middle finger on my chin (a Wangensteen mannerism), and in Dr.
Wangensteen's voice said, "Doctor, why did you . . ." The chief resident turned white; Jack and Don looked stunned. Even I thought
that my words could not possibly have elicited that response.
Unbeknownst to us, Dr. Wangensteen was walking behind us and
had heard the exchange and witnessed my performance. He now
raised his fingers to his chin and, mimicking my mimicking of

him, repeated my question, word for word. The chief resident stammered and gave an inadequate response. Dr. Wangensteen looked at me and smiled, apparently amused by my Wangensteen imitation.

It was Dr. Wangensteen's custom, in our unstructured residency program, to keep a chief resident and one junior resident for four more months on Purple Surgery. It was the prerogative of the chief resident to choose the designated junior resident; none of us wanted four more months with him on Purple Surgery. When I left on a short vacation at the end of June, I felt secure in the belief that the chief resident despised me sufficiently not to choose me, but upon my return, I learned that I was the one chosen. To this day, I do not know how, in a mere week or so, Jack and Don had plagued our chief resident sufficiently to make him forget his antipathy toward me, or if Dr. Wangensteen overruled his choice.

———

Throughout this first year of my training at Minnesota, Daisy taught Freshman English, worked toward her PhD, and cared for Jane with the help of a part-time babysitter. My life partner was also my principal supporter and the keeper of our home. And she was again pregnant.

Looking back, I realize that we worked, one way or another, seven days a week and never believed we were overworked. We were relatively poor but never felt ourselves wanting. We knew we were fortunate, and we were grateful. We were happy in all that we had and in all that we did.

After my abbreviated first year of around nine months, my second year of surgical residency started in July 1961. The major event of that July was the birth of our second daughter, Amy Elizabeth, on July 24. Her arrival was as dramatic as the birth of Jane had been. Jane was born on May 28, 1958, during my internship at Columbia-Presbyterian Medical Center. One evening, Daisy started to bleed profusely from an abruptio placentae (premature separation of the placenta from the uterine wall). I was in the operating room and hurried home. I phoned our obstetrician, Dr. Charles Steer, who was still in the hospital; he said that he would meet us in the obstetrics suite. We lived on the fifth floor of a walk-up several blocks from the hospital. Daisy insisted on putting out the garbage before I helped her down the stairs into a taxi for the short but dramatic ride to the hospital. As I was wheeling Daisy on a gurney into the elevator to the operating rooms, Dr. Virginia Apgar emerged from the elevator, elegantly dressed for a banquet at which she was the speaker. This wonderful woman, a legendary obstetric anesthesiologist and author of the Apgar Score (an index of the baby's health status), reentered the elevator with us and took over. She assured us that we would have a healthy baby. I asked her about her planned evening. She responded that she could talk at another time and that Daisy's and the baby's welfare was of greater importance. Indeed, after an emergency cesarean section by Dr. Steer, with anesthesia by Dr. Apgar, mother and daughter were fine. My debt to these two doctors could only be repaid by emulating them in my own career.

For Amy's birth, we selected the head of the Department of Obstetrics and Gynecology, Dr. Konald Prem, as our obstetrician. He came highly recommended by the house staff, including Jack Bloch, and was the obstetrician who delivered the babies of almost everyone we knew at the university. We believed that Daisy had no anatomical problems that warranted a cesarean section and that it was highly unlikely statistically that she would have a repeat abruptio placenta. Once again, Daisy had a perfectly normal pregnancy, went into labor at the appointed time, and this time had a normal vaginal delivery. However, our baby breathed prematurely in the birth canal and aspirated fluid into her lungs. Amy emerged with aspiration pneumonia and partially collapsed lungs and was placed in a high-oxygen-concentration incubator in the perinatal intensive care unit. We could not hold our child or take her home. We could only pray and wait.

Dr. Prem consulted Dr. Varco and asked him to treat Amy and to decide if the insertion of chest tubes was necessary. Every day, probably three times a day, Varco would come to Amy's enclosed incubator and stare at her intently, counting her respiratory rate, judging her oxygenation by the pinkness of her skin, weighing the options and the risks of further intervention. As an unknown entity in the high-risk postpartum unit, wearing his traditional blue suit and no white coat, he was one day challenged by a floor nurse. He looked at her coldly and told her to go about her work and not to interfere with him doing his. She backed off. At the end of each day of the vigil, Varco would say to me that we should continue to observe but not intercede, other than to supplement Amy's minimal ability to take oral nourishment with an intravenous infusion. After about a week, he said, "She will be all right now. We can stop the IV and let her do it on her own. Tell Mother that she can take her baby home in a few days." He turned, and before I could properly express my gratitude, he was gone.

By taking responsibility for this little being and resisting placing chest tubes or intubating her, Varco may well have saved Amy's life. He could not alleviate the anxiety Daisy and I felt, but in return for our trust he gave us hope and affirmative expectations. I clearly remember standing for hours next to that incubator, encouraging Amy to breathe, wishing I could somehow do it for her. Our second child was a gift of fortune, as was our first. Death had again passed us by.

————

My English Ford Popular with the right-sided drive attracted attention in Minnesota. The Minnesota State driving test examiner at first refused to give me my road test in this vehicle, which required him to sit in the left seat. After some discussion, I convinced him that this configuration was not against the law, explaining that U.S. postal delivery trucks were built in that manner. My test ride was not dramatic: I passed.

When winter came, I donned my Air Force arctic survival suit because the Ford's heater did not work. There also was a loose transmission rod for the accelerator under the hood, which periodically fell off. Once it fell off on a snowy day as I was on my way to work, and I crawled under the car with the hood open to retrieve this essential part of the engine. A passerby stopped and stood there for several minutes watching me grope through the snow before saying, "Lose something?" I did my best imitation of Minnesota laconic and, without looking up, replied, "Nope," continuing in my eventually successful search. The great advantage of this car was that I could always use the hand crank to start it, even after it had been out in subzero weather. Because our garage accommodated only one car, the Ford was always out in the elements, at home and at the university, where residents were not given indoor parking or, for that matter, any parking space at all.

After we acquired Buck, our German shepherd dog who grew to be over 100 pounds, I took particular delight in having him sit in the left front seat of the car. He played his role extremely well, looking straight ahead with an absorbed expression as pedestrians and people in cars gaped at him, the apparent driver. When we stopped at a traffic light with the car windows open, I would hold my hands out of sight on the wheel, turn to Buck and make statements such as, "I told you to make a right turn."

———

My second four-month rotation on Purple Surgery with that problematic chief resident was mostly free of strife. We worked together for the good of our patients. I resolved to help him finish his University of Minnesota tenure in fine fashion, and I often ran interference for him with the two new house staff members of our team. One notable incident, however, involved Dr. Wangensteen. "The Chief" had an extremely old, sick, and incapacitated dog that Mrs. Wangensteen was most attached to. The dog developed painful bleeding hemorrhoids. Dr. Wangensteen asked our resident to operate on the hemorrhoids, winking at him in a way that suggested it would be merciful if the dog did not survive anesthesia. The chief resident did not understand the suggestion, did a successful hemorrhoidectomy, and triumphantly returned the animal to Dr. Wangensteen, who accepted the dog with a look of amazement and consternation.

This rotation on Purple Surgery allowed me to become better acquainted with "The Chief"—his thinking, his vision, his mannerisms, his acerbic comments. As I have alluded to already, there were many unusual people in the surgery department. One of Dr. Wangensteen's sayings was, "I can't tell whether that man is an idiot or a genius. Sometimes the only way I can differentiate between stupidity and genius is that genius has its limits." Dr. Wangensteen also had a profound disregard for the dean of the medical school at the time and on several occasions, at local and national public lectures, he would punctuate his remarks by saying, "The only dean that ever was of any use was Kipling's Gunga Din [pronounced *dean*], the regimental water carrier, for at least he would bring you a drink of water."

"The Chief" was known for his phenomenal memory and photographic recall. At Saturday grand rounds, at complication conferences, or in casual conversation, he would quote from the surgical literature—including the German literature—citing authors, title, year of publication, journal volume, and even the journal page on which the reference could be found. If a resident or student looked at him incredulously, he would, with that trademark twinkle in his eyes, tell him to write down the citation he had just given him and look up the reference in the library.

Dr. Wangensteen needed no reference to the medical literature to offer insights into disease states, often drawing upon his knowledge of Minnesota, his birthplace state. More than one million acres of upper Minnesota bordering on Canada is sheltered federal land comprising the Boundary Waters Canoe Area Wilderness and Voyageurs National Park. This forest and lake country is accessible only by foot and canoe in the nonwinter months, and by skis, snowshoes, and, in restricted areas, snowmobiles in winter. It teems with deer, elk, moose, bears, bobcats, foxes, wolves, and occasional mountain lions. Some Minnesotans, then and now, have chosen to reside in this wilderness, in isolated cabins, living off the land by hunting and fishing. One such recluse was admitted to our service with inanition, lethargy, and mental deterioration. Dr. Wangensteen postulated that this man's terminal disease was caused by eating deer liver. His diagnosis preceded the description of chronic wasting disease in deer by about a decade.

The surgical heroes of the time were all Dr. Wangensteen's friends. We were privileged to be introduced to them by him, whether at the American College of Surgeons annual meeting or when these surgical elites came to visit the University of Minnesota. In this way, I met Drs. Robert M. Zollinger, Robert E. Gross, Thomas E. Starzl, Robert G. Ellison, Lester R. Dragstedt, J. Englebert Dunphy, Denton Cooley, and others, the surgical giants of my youth. The Wangensteen era was not limited in space and time to its progenitor or to the University of Minnesota. For an interval in the mid- to late twentieth century, it included a broader tableau. Zollinger, with his partner Ellison, moved surgical endocrinology

into the twenty-first century with their discovery of the gastrin-
secreting tumor of the pancreas and its metabolic syndrome named
after them. Gross was the first pediatric heart surgeon; Starzl performed the first human liver transplant; Dragstedt was the first to
separate conjoined twins and was noted as an authority on peptic
ulcers; Dunphy made trauma surgery a specialty; and Cooley, the
most technically brilliant cardiac surgeon of that epoch, was the
first to implant an artificial heart. One particular friend of "The
Chief" was Professor Komei Nakayama from Tokyo, Japan, who
delighted in stating, "I am greatest cutting surgeon in the world;
my friend, Dr. Wangensteen, the greatest talking surgeon."

     I have purposely omitted mentioning Dr. Michael E. DeBakey, a
close acquaintance of Dr. Wangensteen, because I loathed DeBakey,
and we became bitter enemies during his lifetime. My first encounter with him was during this second year of my residency. Dr.
Wangensteen asked me to pick up DeBakey at the airport on a Friday evening and drive him to his house. DeBakey was scheduled
to be our guest lecturer at grand rounds the following morning.
I got to the airport with time to spare and waited at the designated arrival gate. In 1961, there was no security system in place.
With several minutes remaining before the scheduled arrival of
DeBakey's flight, I was paged and told to go to the airline counter.
There was DeBakey, seething. He explained that he had arrived in
Chicago from Houston and had run down the tarmac (passengers
still boarded and disembarked from aircraft via a staircase to the
ground), shouting for the next flight to Minneapolis. He found the
flight preceding his scheduled reservation, and, having hand luggage only, boarded the aircraft. He said I should have figured all
that out and met the previous plane. He had called Dr. Wangensteen, who assured him that I was at the airport and told him to
have me paged. I apologized for not being prescient and drove him

to Dr. Wangensteen's house. Throughout the drive, I pointed out the local sights: Minnehaha Falls, the Mississippi River, and so on. DeBakey never responded, never spoke, and never looked at me. At Dr. Wangensteen's house, he left the car without a word. The next day, after DeBakey's lecture, Dr. Wangensteen called me down to the pit of the amphitheater and asked if I would like to drive Dr. DeBakey back to the airport. In a clear, loud voice, to make certain I was heard by DeBakey, I said, "No way." "The Chief" said, "Oh my, oh my," and assigned someone else to the task.

Dr. Wangensteen's technical skills in the operating room were chameleon-like. There were days when his efforts were less than his best, and others, especially when visiting surgeons were present, when they were brilliant. He hated cancer and believed that he could extirpate metastatic intraperitoneal tumor implants and cure the patient even when the tumor had spread beyond the confines of its origin. He would at times send ten or more metastatic foci to pathology, labeled "dome of right diaphragm," "left lobe of liver," "colon," and so on. When he had excised all visible cancer, he often left the operating room, assigning the resident staff to close holes, anastomose bowel, and stop bleeding. Some years later, when Dr. Ward Griffen was the chief resident and I had returned from the laboratory to the clinical services, Dr. Wangensteen asked us why it had taken four hours or so to complete a case involving several bowel resections. Ward answered that for a time we could find only five ends of bowel. "The Chief" gave us his look and his twinkle and said, "Very funny, Dr. Griffen, very funny," and walked on.

Dr. Wangensteen originated what he called the "second-look procedure." Three to six months after a massive cancer resection, especially for colonic and ovarian carcinomas, he would reexplore the patient, looking for recurrences to re-excise and for newly visible tumor implants to remove. He might perform this elective reexploration more than once. The rest of the scientific world scoffed at this "second look," but I believe there were some patients, albeit few, whose lives were saved because of it.

Our outpatient facility, the West Wing Clinic, was in a section of the old Mayo Memorial Building on campus. As a body of four to eight residents and students, we would move with Dr. Wangensteen from room to room seeing follow-up patients and newly referred patients. The patient's chart was in a wooden box on the door to the room. Dr. Wangensteen would briefly peruse the chart before we entered, or one of us would give him an encapsulated patient history. Of course, he remembered each of his prior patients and was always eager to meet and talk to some of them. There was one woman, however, who kept coming back almost weekly with new and insoluble complaints. Dr. Wangensteen did his best to avoid her. When he saw her bulging chart on the door, he walked on and assigned one of us to visit with her. One day we placed the slim chart of a new patient on the door of the examining room in which this particular patient was waiting. "The Chief" eagerly opened the door and, in phalanx fashion, we propelled him into the room before he could escape. He knew he had been trapped. The woman, who had not seen him for months, gushed forth her delight and then followed it up with a litany of complaints. Dr. Wangensteen held up a hand to interrupt and asked her to concentrate on the problem most vexing to her. After some hesitation, she said that she could not sleep at night. Dr. Wangensteen stopped her again and asked her whether she had difficulty in going to sleep or if she woke up during the night. She paused and chose the latter option. Dr. Wangensteen waxed biblical. He took her hand and said, "O, most fortunate of women, when you wake, get out of bed, read, study, improve your mind." With that command, and the rest of us in his wake, he walked out.

Dr. Wangensteen could not shed his farm-boy habits. He went to bed at 9 p.m. and rose well before dawn, and spent the time before coming to the hospital reading and working. His anecdotes often involved his upbringing. When asked why he became a doctor, he would reply with his stock phrase that it beat milking cows at 5 in the morning.

Dr. Wangensteen heard about a dentist in Minneapolis, Dr. Ralph Papermaster, who practiced hypnosis on his patients to augment analgesia. He invited Dr. Papermaster to join the staff to induce postoperative pain control by preoperative hypnosis via a trigger word of posthypnotic suggestion. Dr. Papermaster said he was too busy in his own dental practice but recommended a psychologist who also employed patient hypnosis. Thus, one day the psychologist joined us for rounds. For our first posthypnotic suggestion patient, Dr. Wangensteen selected a middle-aged woman from a Minnesota farm who had come to the university hospital for ulcer surgery the next day. We entered her room in a group consisting of Dr. Wangensteen, the psychologist, and four residents. The patient had just changed into her hospital gown and was sitting up in bed. Dr. Wangensteen told the woman that the psychologist was going to hypnotize her. The psychologist took out a pocket watch and dangled it back and forth by its chain before the patient. He said, over and over, "You are sleepy. You are going to sleep." We stood and watched. The woman was observing us as a group and individually with great curiosity but was not in the least sleepy. Dr. Wangensteen said, "Doctor, she is not going to sleep." The psychologist moved the watch back and forth faster and repeated his incantations with greater urgency. There was no evidence of somnolence on the part of the patient. Dr. Wangensteen said, "Do it! Do it now!" The psychologist began sweating profusely. The woman was looking around, certainly not going to sleep. We were suppressing our mirth. The psychologist was even more uncomfortable as the watch became a blur of movement. Dr. Wangensteen expected his commands to be obeyed and, raising his voice, said, "She is not asleep! Do it now!" At that point, the woman got out of bed, went to the closet and retrieved her clothes. Before she entered the bathroom to dress and leave the hospital, she looked at our entourage and said, "You are all crazy." Looking at Dr. Wangensteen, she said, "And you are the craziest of them all."

✤ 7 ✤

Early Research

The professor's most important role,
I have come to feel, is to create or
help synthesize an atmosphere in
which learning becomes an absorbing,
engaging, and fascinating adventure
in experience.

OWEN H. WANGENSTEEN, *Surgery*
Clinics of North America, 1967

During my second four-month rotation on Purple Surgery, I started my research career at Minnesota. Perhaps Dr. Wangensteen recalled (and he recalled everything) our conversation when I interviewed for a residency position. I stated that I wished to enter his program because I was eager to conduct research as soon as feasible, starting in my residency. Or, possibly, a research project was a test, so to speak, for the junior resident "The Chief" chose for a second, contiguous rotation on Purple Surgery.

I had a demanding schedule. I fulfilled my clinical responsibilities and concurrently worked on two research projects as well as an extracurricular assessment of a newly introduced semisurgical technique. I was generating new information and introducing innovations in patient care—a vast difference from going to school or from learning the tools of the trade for a profession. My surgical

75

education was no longer receptive, merely taking in information, but had become contributory.

The first assignment Dr. Wangensteen gave me was to investigate a remedy for the dumping syndrome, defined by one or more manifestations of nausea, vomiting, diarrhea, flushing, weakness, and the need to lie down, lasting a few minutes to a half hour or so after eating a meal. He had read that individuals with dumping syndrome were relieved by "a pinch of soda," that is, taking sodium bicarbonate, a popular dyspepsia remedy of the day. This syndrome frequently occurred during the era of ulcer surgery. Dumping was seen after subtotal gastrectomies when food, in particular simple carbohydrates, reached the jejunum (upper small intestine) without benefit of being retained in the stomach and the presence of an intervening duodenum (intestinal segment between the stomach and the jejunum). Dr. Wangensteen wanted me to evaluate the bicarbonate observation, because sodium bicarbonate was an alkalizing agent.

I recruited nurses at twenty-five dollars a session to allow me to pass through their nose and the back of their throat into the stomach a self-constructed tube consisting of a plastic conduit with holes at the end and a mercury-weighted condom tip to allow for peristaltic passage through the stomach and duodenum into the proximal jejunum. I checked the position of the tube by X-ray and then, using a room in our intensive-care unit, I infused glucose at acid, neutral, or alkaline pH and recorded the responses of the subject nurses. Indeed, at an alkaline pH, dumping was less frequent and severe than at a neutral or an acid pH. I wrote up the experiment and published it. Nothing came of this finding and no more on this phenomenon was reported in the literature. As it happens, the specific mechanism for the dumping effect still remains unknown.

My other assignment from Dr. Wangensteen was to initiate

Mohs's paste surgery at the university. Dr. Frederic E. Mohs, a Wisconsin surgeon, had developed a paste to be applied to skin cancers in cosmetically sensitive areas where wide-margin resections would be disfiguring—for example, the nose. The paste consists of a tissue-killing substance, a fixative, and a glue to hold the paste together. After the paste is applied, within forty-eight hours, the fixed tissue is bloodlessly excised, sectioned, stained, and examined under a microscope. Edges of the resection containing residual tumor are immediately retreated, re-excised, and so on, until the area is tumor-free. I extended this methodology in order to pursue tumors beyond the confines of a safe primary resection. For example, I treated a patient with a basal-cell carcinoma that had destroyed the bridge of her nose and was penetrating the frontal sinuses and moving through the skull into the frontal cranial cavity. I treated this tumor with Mohs's paste applications but waited longer than forty-eight hours before resecting the fixed tissue. By waiting, I avoided a spinal fluid leak as I penetrated the meninges into the frontal brain cavity containing cerebrospinal fluid. This lovely lady survived to live tumor-free. Some years later, I saw her with her daughter at a performance of the traveling Metropolitan Opera Company. She had a plastic nose prosthesis attached to her glasses that blended into her face. She appeared to be healthy and happy. The Mohs's procedure not only saved her life but enhanced its quality.

During the early 1960s, Dr. Wangensteen, his laboratory, and his clinical service experimented with gastric cooling for bleeding gastric and duodenal ulcers, and with gastric freezing to cure the ulcer diathesis. An oral gastric balloon was placed inside the stomach and attached to inflow and outflow conduits through which a coolant was circulated. Depending on the temperature set for the coolant, the stomach was made extremely cold or was actually frozen. Because the cooled stomach constricted bleeding vessels, this therapy was often successful. The frozen stomach was intended to injure acid-secreting parietal cells to prevent gastric acid output when the stomach was thawed. This procedure rarely worked, and occasionally a frozen stomach ruptured, requiring emergency surgery.

During my time on Purple Surgery, I completed one other independently initiated, minor clinical project on the postoperative use of tracheal stimulation, whose outcome was published in the journal *Surgery*. In order to avoid pneumonia after general anesthesia, patients must cough and breathe deeply to open collapsed air-exchange pockets in the lungs. However, coughing after surgery is painful and many patients resist, forcing direct stimulation of the trachea by the medical staff to elicit a vigorous cough response. For this procedure, a doctor or a nurse inserts a small catheter through the nose, which is quite distressing to the patient. Instead, for my project, with a needle stick in the neck, I placed a catheter directly into the trachea, which could be left in place without discomfort and manipulated by the medical staff when necessary to induce coughing, at far less distress to the patient.

My months on Purple Surgery were not all work. I made time for my growing family, and for physical exercise. And I started a highly pleasurable position as house doctor at the university's concert facility at Northrop Auditorium for more than twenty years of performances. Shortly after our arrival in Minnesota, I attempted to purchase tickets to dance and orchestral events at Northrop Auditorium. I was offered two seats with a partially blocked view in the rear of the theater at what seemed to me at the time an exorbitant price. I rejected these seats and went to see the theater director; I informed him that I was a first-year resident at the University Hospital and hoped that he could do better for me. By a stroke of luck, the previous house doctor had resigned that morning. The director asked if I wanted two eighteenth-row orchestra aisle seats to all performances—free. I thought, "This is more like it!" I agreed and became the longest-serving house doctor in the history of Northrop Auditorium. When I could not attend a performance, I readily found other doctors to take my place.

In the 1960s, the Metropolitan Opera went on the road to perform in several cities, including Minneapolis, after its regular New York season. At times, the opera played bait and switch with its headliners. It advertised stars such as Luciano Pavarotti, but at the performance, the understudy played the role after it was announced that the star was "indisposed." As house doctor, Daisy and I went to all seven performances during Metropolitan Opera Week. I worked all day, traded my night call, and was tired the next day, but it was worth it. I went backstage to attend to minor problems, such as removing a splinter from the buttock of a ballerina who had been required to slide across the wooden stage floor during her dance scene.

I have always been an opera buff, and I was thrilled to be able to observe the stars of opera from backstage. I met Renata Tebaldi in her dressing room with her personal maid between acts of *Tosca*. She was all concentration and no levity, the epitome of the prima donna. Franco Corelli, a splendid tenor, had to pet his poodle, held out to him by his wife, before each act. On the other hand, the exemplar of relaxation was Richard Tucker, one of the greatest tenors of all time. He stood in the wings, calmly sorting and reading his mail as the stage manager, with increasing urgency, said, "Two minutes, Mr. Tucker," "One minute, Mr. Tucker," and "Thirty seconds, Mr. Tucker." At "Five seconds, Mr. Tucker," Mr. Tucker handed his mail to the stage manager, gave me and others standing there a nod and a smile, and ran out onto the stage in tears, singing a grief-stricken lamentation.

The Wangensteen surgery residency consisted of two years postinternship of clinical rotations. These rotations were followed

by two or more years in a basic science laboratory while taking
courses for a PhD in surgery and/or a PhD or MS in a basic science such as biochemistry. The two final years of clinical training
were the senior and chief years of residency. As already mentioned,
the different clinical services were named after colors, for reasons I
never understood.

When my time on Purple Surgery was drawing to an end, Dr.
Wangensteen invited me to come into his laboratory after I completed my second year of junior residency. I politely refused, stating
that I was not interested in working in gastric physiology, fascinating though it was. No one had ever turned down a coveted invita-
tion by "The Chief" to come into his laboratory. He sweetened the
offer by promising me the position of head of the laboratory after
my first laboratory year, a title that essentially guaranteed an offer
of a staff position after completion of residency training. Again, I
politely refused. At this point, he asked me what I was interested in.
I told him I wanted to explore cholesterol metabolism and atherosclerotic coronary artery disease, and that I would probably choose
to follow a career in cardiovascular, not gastrointestinal, surgery. He
responded that all he really knew about cholesterol was that if you
painted it on the back of a newt, the animal would develop a cancer. He told me to work with Dr. Varco but to come and see him
after my next four-month rotation. I asked Dr. Aust, who was in
charge of the residency program, to place me on Dr. Varco's Orange
Surgery service starting in October 1961, and Dr. Varco approved
my request.

———

I ended my eight-month Purple Surgery sojourn after one year in
Minnesota, thoroughly indoctrinated into the unique Wangen-
steen residency training program, and a full-fledged Minnesotan.
Daisy and I lived in a house, had friends in the community, found

out that there was no gourmet Scandinavian restaurant in the Twin Cities, planned to go up north to canoe and hike in the wilderness, and learned to say "you betcha" for "I agree," or "it is my intention," or a simple "yes," as well as "uff da" as an exclamation for just about anything.

Varco's Surgery Service

Tough love.

BILL MILLIKEN AND CHAR MEREDITH,
Tough Love, 1968

The rotation on Orange Surgery offered me many insights into the complex character of Richard Varco. Dr. Varco was a technical marvel in the operating room, as well as a physician, scholar, innovative thinker, teacher, examiner, academic, curmudgeon, family man, hunter, gardener, and cook—and my friend-to-be. He was a true general surgeon and few were his equal in operative skill. His expertise encompassed head and neck, breast, thoracic, gastrointestinal, colorectal, cardiovascular, peripheral vascular, and endocrine surgery, with some urologic and gynecologic procedures as well. His technical skills were legendary, and surgeons, in particular Walt Lillehei and the other surgeons struggling to perform heart operations in the new discipline of cardiovascular surgery, called upon him to assist and to teach them. He performed surgery with extraordinary delicacy and minimal blood loss though his hands were huge; they were the hands of a Montana rancher and manual laborer. He once looked at my relatively small hands (I wear size 6½ surgical gloves) and said, "What do you hope to do with those little things?" I responded, "To operate in areas you can't even get into with those things," indicating his hands. He wore size 8½ surgical gloves; most surgeons wear size 7 or 7½.

I was soon to be tested by Varco—in the operating room, on the wards—on how I thought and reasoned. In addition, he wanted to see how resilient I was. Many residents feared the Orange Surgery rotation, but I welcomed it. Varco was worth emulating. I wanted this apprenticeship with the man who had the fabled reputation of being the best of the best.

My operating room apprenticeship with Varco started in earnest with a patent ductus arteriosus (PDA) repair in a tiny baby. A PDA is failure of closure of a vestigial conduit between the left pulmonary artery and the aorta. If left unchecked it would lead to heart failure. In order to avoid life-threatening bleeding, this vessel needs to be divided between clamps with the ends carefully oversewn before the removal of the clamps. Varco allowed me to perform the procedure under his careful supervision. I divided the ductus and meticulously, with a very fine suture, made a running closure from right to left, sewing from the left side of the patient with my right hand. On completion of the first row of the closure, Varco asked me how I had planned to run the suture back to its origin to provide a second row of closure before tying the retaining knots. I responded that I would now sew backhand, or that I would come over to his side of the operating room table to again sew forehand. He responded that I would do neither, that I would stay where I was and sew forehand with my left hand. So, I did. So, I learned.

Varco's care of patients outside the operating room was as meticulous and successful as his work in the operating room. Every case received his individual attention. He examined the parameters of pathology and therapy well beyond the conventional. He trusted only a few internists and cardiologists and, for the most part, was his patient's physician as well as his or her surgeon. During his own training, he had spent a year in radiology and he relied on his own readings of X-rays, especially the newly introduced arteriographic studies. From Varco I adopted my lifetime concept of caring for the total patient, heeding the advice of a few select consultants, and, above all, taking responsibility for all that occurred during my tenure of care for a patient. In my teaching of this concept since that time, I instruct my residents that if a patient falls out of bed, or has an equally unforeseen event, this event did not "just happen" but was the resident's fault.

Richard Varco was a scholar in multiple aspects of surgery and the medical sciences. He read voraciously, though in spite of my later urgings, I don't believe he ever read a novel. He considered nonscientific writing frivolous. He told me that he had tried reading poetry on several occasions and that he did not understand the medium. His hero was Albert Einstein, whom he quoted liberally.

Throughout his surgical career, he attended the principal surgical meetings. At a single plenary session meeting format (i.e., where there are no concurrent sessions), such as that of the American Surgical Association, he would be in a front-row seat every day at the appointed hour for the first paper, and he would listen to every paper until the end of the day's session. Other surgeons at these meetings (including myself) would walk out of the session to chat with friends over coffee, return to the hotel room, or go sightseeing when a paper outside of the surgeon's purview was being presented. Not Varco. He listened, commenting at times on the presentation and judging the validity of the contents of a paper and the intellectual credentials of the presenter.

Varco was well known and widely consulted for his innovative thinking. His forte was taking a clinical problem or a research concept and dissecting and analyzing its myriad ramifications with a freshness of thought and a novel approach. Often the same question posed at different times resulted in varied but equally cogent responses. A visit to Varco's office for a patient consultation or discussion of an innovative concept was never disappointing. Such occasions almost always generated a new insight or perspective.

He was the best of teachers and the worst. In the operating room, he taught by example and by allowing graduated responsibility. Out of the operating room, he employed the Socratic method of questioning, debating, and reanalyzing, always moving to the next level of cognitive insight and never letting his disciple rest on his intellectual accomplishments. Praise from Varco was, essentially, nonexistent. When I did something extremely well in the operating room and was stupid enough to fish for a compliment, I was given a grunt and told, "I can teach a monkey to operate." When I was satisfied with my reasoning capability, I was given a grunt and taken onward to a previously unexplored plane of perception. He taught that growth of mind and the pleasure of thought were the true eternal verities.

On the other hand, Varco was dismissive of residents he did not wish to work with. During my first Orange Surgery rotation, I was paired with another junior resident named Bob who Varco disdained. He never scheduled Bob for the operating room. Once when I told Bob to take my place in the operating room while I did his ward chores, consults, and the like, Bob came looking for me within minutes to tell me that Varco had asked him to leave the operating room and for me to take his place. When I arrived, Varco said, "I'll decide who will scrub."

Varco had the reputation of being the toughest and meanest American Board of Surgery examiner in its history. He held the prestigious post of board examiner for many years and was extremely proud of this rigorous task. After completing medical school, five years of clinical training in surgery, one year of practicing surgery, and passing the written board examination, a board candidate would face the oral examination and, possibly, Varco.

He believed that certain individuals, even at this advanced stage of professional training, should not be certified as surgeons, and that to do so would be a disservice to the discipline and to future patients. At the same time, if he believed in a board candidate, he would become that person's champion. I took many simulated board exams prior to the real one, where, of course, I could not draw Varco as an examiner because we were from the same institution. I took these practice exams whenever there was a leisure moment—in Varco's office, for example, and especially on airplanes. Varco and I would sit together when we flew to meetings. I would take out some piece of work or make the mistake of opening a novel. Varco would growl at me, "Put that away. We are going to have a board exam." When it came to my actual examination, except for the questions of one neurosurgeon, the sessions were actually enjoyable and remarkably easy.

In Varco's perception of academia and the university, both the concept and the institution were holy. During his active career, and in his retirement, he made many enemies in academia and at the University of Minnesota. A few he earned because of his difficult disposition, but most were put off by his high principles, his dedication to knowledge, and his belief that academia was a sanctuary for higher learning and freedom of expression. I shared his sentiments but would, on occasion, make disparaging comments about events at the university. He would stop me and state that my anger and disappointment should be directed toward the temporary inhabitants of positions of power—deans, vice presidents, presidents—and not toward the institution itself. For him, a university was an eternal ideal, the habitat of knowledge, thought, and reflection.

Varco was the epitome of a curmudgeon. Twenty years my senior, his persona was old-fashioned, blunt, and off-putting. His general demeanor of hostility served him well. Few people would risk displeasing him; most wanted to avoid him or to anticipate and fulfill his wishes. On social occasions, he displayed an alter ego of gentlemanly courtesy and self-deprecation. A poor boy from a ranch in Montana, he had earned a small fortune. Yet he wore the same shiny blue suit most of his life. (None of us knew if it was one blue suit or two interchangeable suits to allow for cleaning.) He usually also wore a blue shirt, often with a tear in the pocket, and a stained blue tie. He never wore the attending surgeon's white coat. In the coldest weather, he did not wear (or own?) an overcoat. He was quite stout, and it was said (behind his back) that he wore his overcoat subcutaneously. One fall, after unsuccessfully hunting mountain goats on horseback, he decided he had to lose weight in order to try again the following year. I estimate that he lost about fifty pounds. He pleated the waist of his suit pants and made extra holes in his belt, which almost fit twice around his now much smaller waist. I asked him why he did not purchase another suit, or at least new pants and belt. He said he would only regain the weight after the fall hunting season. He lost weight, successfully shot a mountain goat, and reexpanded to his original girth.

One day, Varco was highly displeased with the care of a patient on the intensive-care unit. He severely upbraided the nurse in charge, punctuating his harsh criticisms with the term "girlie." When she could no longer endure his tirade, the nurse started to cry and screamed back, "You are nothing but a sexist." I was not present for this encounter but was told that Varco stopped his diatribe, looked reflective, and responded, "I don't know what that is, girlie, but it sounds pretty good to me." Later on, he cornered me and asked, "What is a sexist?" I told him that it was not a compliment.

Almost everyone in the Department of Surgery in the 1960s had large families. Richard Varco had the largest, with eight children. Joe Aust, with seven children, was once discreetly asked by Dr. Wangensteen, who had three children, whether his wife was a Catholic. Joe responded that she was a "very hot Protestant." Varco's wife was Catholic; I have no knowledge whether her religious beliefs influenced the size of their family. When one of the Varco's daughters was in kindergarten, the teacher asked the children in the class to express "a happy thought." The little Varco girl said, "I am pregnant." The teacher, taken aback, told the child that she was not pregnant and asked why that statement was a happy thought. The girl responded that on that morning, "Mommy did not come down for breakfast and did not feel well. When she came down the stairs, she said to Daddy, 'I am pregnant,' and Daddy said, 'That's a happy thought.'" His family was sacrosanct to Varco. He treated his wife, Louise, with deference, and I believe his children, especially the boys, with the same "tough love" reserved for his favorite pupils.

From childhood, Varco hunted and, once he could afford them, collected expensive, hand-made hunting guns. His hunting clothing, contrary to his daily wear, was meticulously selected and utilitarian; cost was not spared. He hunted birds, deer, mountain goats, and more, but he was not a trophy hunter and never went big-game hunting in foreign lands. He told me that, especially as he grew older, the thrill of hunting was sitting in a duck blind and watching the sun come up, walking across a native prairie of high grass, or being in mountains blazing with fall colors. He said he often would sight a quarry along his gun barrel, lower his gun, and marvel at the animal free in nature.

Varco cooked and made sausage from game he killed. He baked his own bread. In the spring and summer, he gardened. He raised flowers as well as vegetables. He stated that he raised enough of a particular vegetable, such as carrots, to feed his family as well as the rabbits.

It was during my first rotation on Orange Surgery that my mentor/mentee relationship with Dr. Varco started to evolve into a lifelong friendship, and he and I became comfortable with my addressing him as "Richard." The friendship grew ever stronger and lasted until his death in 2004. Our relationship was based on trust, respect, and enjoyment of each other's company and conversation, as well as a mutual affection never verbally expressed. Although my relationship with Varco was recognized by my peers as eminently profitable for my career, few, if any, envied my friendship with this unique, acerbic giant of American surgery.

The initiation of our new relationship might have started with an argument. In November 1961, I was scrubbed with Varco on a vascular procedure in the upper thigh of a patient. He asked me the name of a particular muscle. I was well prepared for this case, and I knew the anatomy. I responded, "The adductor magnus." He said I was wrong and named another regional muscle. I said that I was certain that it was the adductor magnus. He asked me why I would blatantly stand there and contradict him. I replied that this matter was not a contest of wills or opinions, but that the muscle in question always had been, was, and would remain the adductor magnus. In essence, it was what it was. He scowled and stomped out of the operating room, and returned with the operating room desk surgical atlas, a book with poor illustrations that could be interpreted as favoring his naming of the muscle in question. Nevertheless, I stood my ground. He scowled at me for a long time and said, "I'll be damned. You are self-righteous and arrogant." We spoke no more that day.

I was free that evening by about 9 p.m. and called Daisy to tell her I would be home late. I went to the library, pulled out the best anatomical texts and atlases, hand-copied their description of the adductor magnus muscle, its origin, and its insertion, accompanied by my reproductions of the drawings in the atlases. (There were no copying machines in 1961.) I then hand-made three individual copies of this information, which proved, without a doubt, that I was right and that Varco was wrong. I put one copy under Varco's office door, slipped one into his operating room locker, and, at midnight, headed for his home on the East River Road. When I got there, I parked in the street, prowled to his back door (the one he used to enter his garage in the morning), and slipped the third copy under the door. Throughout all my harried activity, his dog barked furiously, snapping at the door between us.

The next morning, I was scrubbed when Varco entered the operating room. He said nothing about the notes. Our conversation was confined to the surgery. Later that afternoon, he said only, "Why three copies?" I answered, "So that you won't forget it." In this episode of the adductor magnus, I was who I was. And Varco, in some strange way, being who he was, respected me and responded by trying to work me to death or break me in some other manner over the next three months. At the end of the rotation, he made me a present of Edward Pernkopf's two-volume anatomical atlas, clearly the best atlas of anatomy ever illustrated. Neither of us knew then that Pernkopf was a high-level Nazi who had based his anatomical dissections on the bodies of concentration camp victims.

As I survived the rotation, Varco incrementally increased my surgical responsibilities. Close to the end of the rotation, however, I committed a bad error. About midnight, I was to cut down on the brachial vein and insert an IV line in our open-heart patient for the next morning. I cut down and threaded the IV catheter into the brachial artery instead, a fact I became aware of when there was no flow down the IV tubing, but rather a pumping red column coming from the patient. I called Aldo Castaneda, the chief resident. I was surprised when he told me to call and tell Varco. That was wrong of him. He should have come in and helped me correct my mistake, as I would have done were I the chief resident. I called Varco as instructed and woke him; he listened, said, "Fix it," and hung up. I spent the next few hours alone, fixing my mistake. By

5 a.m., I had a good venous line in the brachial vein and a repaired brachial artery with a strong palpable pulse at the wrist. It was now time to go to the operating room to cut Styrofoam baffles for the mitral valve repair that morning, followed by rounds at 6 a.m., and scrubbing in by 7 a.m. Sleep would have to wait. Aldo was displeased that I had been so foolish as to mistake the artery for the vein, and probably unhappy that, without begging for his help, I was able to repair my mistake. Varco never said a word about it.

I trusted Varco with our daughter Amy when she was born with a partially collapsed lung. During that same period, I also trusted him to repair our daughter Jane's branchial cleft cyst, a neck cyst connecting with the oral cavity and draining mucus. The repair went well.

With the end of my tenure on Orange Surgery, I had completed only seventeen months of the twenty-four months of an orthodox junior residency in surgery. I was, however, ready to move on. I felt comfortable in the operating room and in taking care of patients. I had innovative thoughts ready for exploration. The laboratory beckoned.

✤ 9 ✤

Laboratory Founded

*In the lively leaven of an atmosphere
fostering inquiry, no one was afraid
to come forward with a novel idea, no
matter how strange or unfamiliar it
may have sounded. The stages of a new
idea are multiple. Many are stillborn.
But every new suggestion deserves
at least a trial of being blown upon
in the hope that there may be sparks
in the ashes.*

OWEN H. WANGENSTEEN, *Journal of
the American Medical Association,*
1968

I went to see Dr. Wangensteen in February 1962. I told him that I
wanted to leave the clinical services in March to start my laboratory
years and that I would complete my second-year residency training
when I returned to the clinical services. I expressed my belief that
I had learned a great deal and had done a considerable amount of
surgery in my seventeen months of junior residency. I also pointed
out that a basic science course I wanted to take for my PhD degree
would start in March. In the fluid residency program of the time,
this individualization of training was not uncommon. It was said
by outsiders, often despairingly, that the residency training program

at Minnesota was an inscrutable tunnel: people entered at one end and emerged seven to ten years later from the other end as surgeons and academics, but that all that happened within the tunnel was a mystery. There were no national standards at that time for the conduct of, and prescribed surgical procedures for, a surgical residency program, other than five years of clinical training.

Dr. Wangensteen readily granted my request to leave the clinical services. He asked me once again, pro forma, to enter his laboratory, expecting my polite refusal. We were then ready to move on. I told him that I wanted to have my own laboratory. He replied that a resident had never had his own laboratory (indeed, no one did in future years), but that he would grant this wish as well. He said that he would provide me with a twenty-thousand-dollar budget (a huge sum in 1962) for one year and twenty thousand dollars for a second year if I was unable to secure outside funding. He called Dr. Ivan D. Frantz, a professor of biochemistry and a lipid expert, requesting that he serve as my PhD adviser. Finally, he said that I should talk with Dr. Varco, who commanded research space and additional funds, stating that I seemed to have established a favorable relationship with him. Dr. Wangensteen invited me to come and tell him about my work at any time, emphasizing that this was not necessary but purely voluntary. He wished me success.

A short time later, the then-current head of Dr. Wangensteen's laboratory called me and said that it was his job to know about every resident's research project. I had never trusted this person. Varco did not trust him, and I was certain that the basis of his request was not only invalid but also unknown to Dr. Wangensteen, who would not have permitted this inquiry. If this resident thought my ideas worthwhile, I believed that he would steal them. I agreed to meet with him. I spun out a research project in cholesterol metabolism with no relationship to my actual plans, a concept that, upon any serious reflection, was doomed to fail. He listened, real-

ized the inevitable failure inherent in this project, and said that my
idea was great and encouraged me to pursue it vigorously. He was
convinced that I was not going to be a future competitor. There are
those who climb the ladder of success ignoring others, those who
help others up a rung or two, and those who try to kick others off.

I went to see Varco and told him my actual plans in detail. He
liked them. I informed him of my conversation with Dr. Wangensteen. Varco offered me a small laboratory space, a windowless area
the size of a storage closet. He asked me what equipment I needed.
I said that the most expensive item was a scintillation counter, but
that I would have free use of one in Dr. Frantz's laboratory. I said
that the tiny laboratory space was sufficient for my needs but that
the stone benchtops and the standard exhaust hood were not. I
would be using radioactive $C14$ and $H3$ isotopes. If they spilled on
the stone, they would be absorbed and could not be removed. Also,
the hood's filter could not handle radioactive substances. Varco
asked me what needed to be done. I told him that the stone tops
had to be covered with stainless steel and the hood replaced by a
radioactivity-sensitive one. He purchased these items and had them
installed. Indeed, my laboratory was the first in the medical school
to have stainless-steel workbenches and a specialized hood for protection from radiation dissemination.

In March 1962, my dream of many years became a reality. I had
my own laboratory. I was free to pursue concepts, create experiments, execute the requisite work, analyze the findings, move
toward a goal, learn from errors, and publish my results. My time
was my own to allocate; I had no one to report to, no one to
explain or justify my work to. I had time for contemplation. Orig-
inating ideas and turning them into the reality of practical application were mine to explore. I dived into these pristine waters of
creativity like a creature of that sea celebrating a homecoming or,
more accurately, a birth.

Over the next two years, 1962–64, the earliest years of my independent research, I conceived an idea and explored its ramifications. Working from hypothesis through experiment, I came up with the original concept of the partial ileal bypass for hypercholesterolemia. I established new basic science data that has since become part of the textbook literature in gastrointestinal physiology and biochemistry. I performed what is today termed *translational research*: I took a concept through animal and clinical testing into patient care as a new therapeutic alternative in a field that, about fifteen years later, I defined as metabolic surgery. Over subsequent years, I contributed several research innovations that were improvements on, or expansions of, prior work or procedures. I provided additions to established knowledge or applications—the usual step-by-step progress in science and medicine. I worked with many others, combining perspectives and experience to formulate hypotheses and create new inventions. I believe, however, that my unique idea resulting in the partial ileal bypass operation may well represent my single best scientific contribution.

In 1962, there were no effective or safe drugs to lower cholesterol, which had been identified as a major risk factor for the ever-increasing epidemic of atherosclerotic cardiovascular disease, the progenitor of heart attacks, strokes, and peripheral vascular disease. The best cholesterol-lowering therapy available was dietary modification, with reductions in the intake of total fats and cholesterol.

Circulating cholesterol consists of cholesterol synthesized by the body, primarily in the liver, and of ingested cholesterol. Liver-secreted bile contains high concentrations of cholesterol, about 60 percent of which is reabsorbed in the small intestine. This circulation is known as the enterohepatic cholesterol cycle. Bile acids are derived from cholesterol in the liver for secretion into the bile and about 90 percent of the bile acids are reabsorbed in the small intestine. This complementary process is known as the enterohepatic

bile acid cycle. In essence, humans use the same bile acids for emul-
sification of fats for breakfast, lunch, and dinner. The cholesterol
and bile acids enterohepatic pathways represent the body's cholesterol exit mechanism. The balance achieved by cholesterol intake
and production with its excretion determines the blood cholesterol
concentration, which can range from low (good) to high (bad) levels.

I reasoned that removing the appropriate segment of the small
intestine from contact with the flow of ingested foodstuffs and gastric and intestinal secretions would result in interference with the
enterohepatic cholesterol and bile acid cycles. This interference
would then, in turn, decrease cholesterol bile acid absorption and
reabsorption, while increasing cholesterol and bile acid excretion.
I further reasoned that this direct drain of body cholesterol, plus
the indirect drain of body cholesterol by forcing its conversion to
replenish bile acids, would result in a compensatory increase in
body cholesterol synthesis. At what level would the engendered
increase in cholesterol turnover be reflected in the plasma cholesterol and in the cholesterol concentrations of the other body
cholesterol pools? In other words, at what level would all this metabolic cholesterol activity reach equilibrium in the blood cholesterol, a progenitor indicator of atherosclerosis?

My reading of existing literature informed me that Byers, Friedman, and Gunning had shown that cholesterol is absorbed exclusively in the small intestine, and preferentially in the distal (lower)
half. Lack and Weiner had also demonstrated that bile acids were
preferentially absorbed in the distal small intestine. These were the
facts that were known about cholesterol and bile acid gut metabolism. No one had thought of regulating blood cholesterol levels
by intestinal exclusion, thereby reducing its propensity for eliciting
atherosclerotic cardiovascular disease. As a surgeon, I hypothesized
that bypassing the distal ileum, that is, performing a partial ileal

bypass, would influence cholesterol metabolism and thereby miti-
gate atherosclerosis. I started with three experiments whose results I
would eventually publish.

This work involved sequential hypothesis testing in rabbits,
pigs, and humans. These experiments showed that partial ileal
bypass significantly decreased cholesterol absorption and the aver-
age blood cholesterol level. I studied seven human volunteers who
had previously undergone a partial ileectomy for causes other than
carcinoma—for example, incarcerated hernia (an abdominal wall
defect with entrapped bowel)—and compared them to seven vol-
unteer control subjects. These affirmative determinations were
made years after the seven ileectomy patients had undergone their
resection, indicating that the ileal exclusion lipid effect was lasting.

In the beginning of this study, I worked alone in the laboratory.
For the initial rabbit series, I came to the hospital early and checked
on my animals. According to my work schedule, I prepared the C14
cholesterol emulsions and fed by stomach tube gavage the selected
rabbits. I took blood samples from an ear vein and stored the specimens for analysis. On animal surgery days, I transported the rabbits
to my little room of a laboratory, prepared them for surgery, did
my own anesthesia, performed the partial ileal bypasses by myself,
and sat and warmed the animals with a heating blanket until they
were alert and could be returned to their cages. In the afternoon,
I usually turned biochemist and extracted the cholesterol from
the blood specimens, using a spectrophotometer to determine the
milligrams per sample. I measured the C14 radioactivity in a scintillation spectrometer, made available to me in Dr. Frantz's vast laboratory across the hall. Today's spectrometers measure up to 250
samples automatically and provide the researcher with a computer
readout of results. I had to measure each sample, and its duplicate,
individually by hand, allowing an hour for the radioactivity count
to be completed, and my recording the beta particles emitted and

registered on the screen of the counter in my laboratory notebook. To complete a test run, doing one sample at a time, often took me until midnight or longer.

Performing the initial pig experiments was the hardest. The animals were housed at the College of Veterinary Medicine on the St. Paul campus of the university, referred to at that time as the farm campus. The animals were young, spotted Poland China pigs, weighing about thirty pounds each. Again, I did everything myself. For surgery, I loaded the animals onto the back of a pickup truck and drove them from the animal pens to the building containing the animal operating rooms. Preparation, anesthesia, surgery, and postoperative care were all up to me. Operating room assistance was not available.

One series of events in December 1962 stands out in my memory. It had been snowing all day. I had been operating from the morning on and when, after dark, I placed the animals in the bed of the pickup to return them to the animal storage building, I wore only a scrub suit. The cold air combined with the pig danders that covered me gave me respiratory tightness close to an asthma attack. When I came home, Daisy said I smelled like a pig. I took a long shower and scrubbed very hard. Daisy said I still smelled like a pig. The next morning, I visited my pigs. Two were missing. I asked the attendant where they were. He replied, "They et 'em," pointing to the other pigs in the pen. Indeed, I found the hoofs and snouts of the missing pigs in the straw of the large pen I had been assigned. Apparently, the pigs that had been operated on earlier that day, and those not undergoing surgery that day, ate the pigs returning weakened from surgery.

In 1962 and 1963, there were no computerized record-keeping systems or data banks. To obtain information about the patients in the original retrospective patient series I had to consult catalogs and then search through row upon row of dusty patient records in the long-term storage room. After that, I would contact the patients and obtain their consent for the study, administer the radioactive C14 cholesterol in a butter tidbit, and calculate the cholesterol absorption curves and cholesterol levels. After the exhaustive work of searching the records, the rest seemed relatively easy.

The final section of the 1964 paper based on this testing consisted of the first clinical report of partial ileal bypass in four familial hypercholesterolemic patients—patients with congenital, genetically determined, extremely high plasma (blood) cholesterol levels (hyperlipidemia). I performed the world's first partial ileal bypass for hyperlipidemia on May 29, 1963, when I was a junior resident under the protection of Varco. In these partial ileal bypass patients, cholesterol absorption by the C14 cholesterol test was decreased by 40 percent to 50 percent, and the plasma cholesterol level by 30 percent to 60 percent.

With the publication of that paper, partial ileal bypass became a clinical entity. There are no coauthors on the 1964 *Circulation* paper, because I had no coworkers. This paper may indeed be my cardinal contribution to the medical literature. It was extremely well received at Minnesota and elsewhere; however, there were notable exceptions.

I submitted an abstract with these results to the American Heart Association (AHA). The paper was accepted for a major session presentation at the annual meeting of the society in Los Angeles in October 1963. In the audience was Dr. Louis Katz, a renowned cardiologist and atherosclerosis researcher from Chicago with a reputation for being caustic, condescending, savage, insulting, and downright mean, in addition to being brilliant, respected, feared, and influential in the AHA and at the National Institutes of Health (NIH). When I completed my talk, which ended with a discussion of the first four partial ileal bypass patients, Katz got to his feet and castigated me for several minutes, calling my work unethical

and the worst thing he had ever heard since the "Nazi concentration camps." This comment by an American Jew to a fellow Jew, a
Holocaust survivor, shocked me. I was furious and, in spite of being
a mere resident, I struck back at the professor, defending my work
and ending my statement with a contemptuous comment about
Katz's own research work that used chickens as human surrogates.
A science reporter for the *Los Angeles Times* heard this exchange,
and Katz and I were featured in his paper the next day, under a
headline proclaiming, "Chicken Debate at the AHA."

I felt a tremendous letdown. I had naively expected to be lauded
for my seminal work to lower cholesterol and, in the process,
ameliorate atherosclerosis, the cause of heart attacks and strokes.
Innocently, I anticipated instant recognition and acceptance by
the fellows of the AHA. I had envisioned comments praising this
innovative work and questions as to where I believed lipid/athero-
sclerosis research should now be directed. If there were any such
thoughts in the minds of my audience, the dismissive, condemning
statement of Louis Katz inhibited all further discussion. After his
attack and my rebuttal, there was silence. Katz, in a huff, walked out
with his entourage. I sat down and pretended to listen to the next
speaker.

The annual meeting of the American College of Surgeons (ACS)
was scheduled to start in San Francisco a few days after the AHA
meeting. I rented a car and drove up fabled Highway 1 to San Francisco through Santa Barbara, Big Sur, and Monterey. I checked into
my inexpensive hotel in the evening. Before 7 a.m., I was in the
lobby of the ACS headquarters hotel, the Fairmont, placing a call to
Dr. Wangensteen's room. He was an early riser and within minutes
of my call came down to the lobby to meet with me. We sat behind
one of the huge potted palms in the lobby of the Fairmont and I
related my experience in Los Angeles with Dr. Katz.

Dr. Wangensteen listened attentively. When I mentioned Katz,

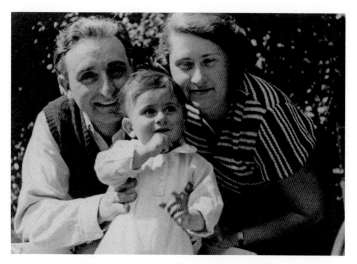

With my parents, Andor and Renée, in Vienna in 1932, the year I was born.

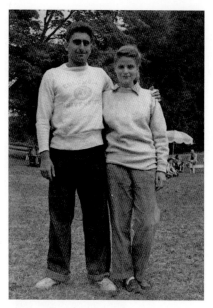

With Daisy on a picnic in 1952, two years before our marriage.

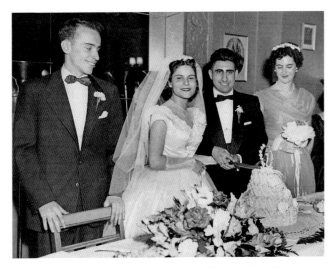

Our wedding in New York, 1954.

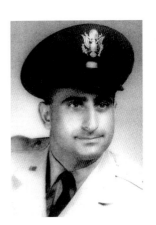

Flight Surgeon, Captain
USAF, SAC, 1958.

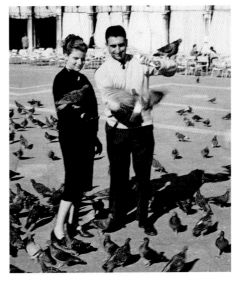

On leave in Venice, 1958.

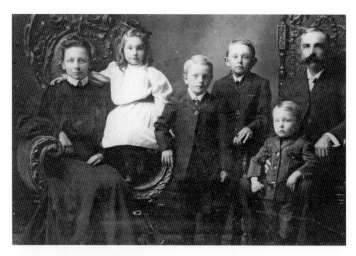

Owen Wangensteen (center) with his family, circa 1905. Mother Hannah is at left and father Ove at right. Courtesy of the University of Minnesota Department of Surgery.

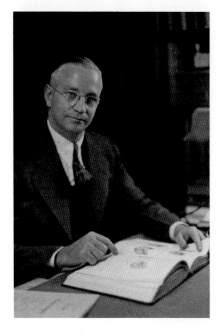

Wangensteen the doctoral student, circa 1930. Courtesy of the University of Minnesota Archives.

My first clinical experiment at the University of Minnesota, 1960.

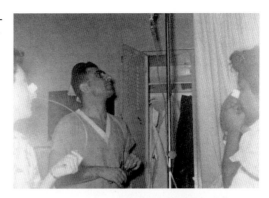

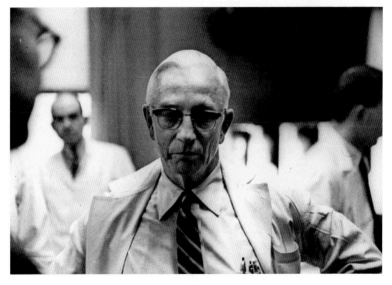

Owen Wangensteen, around the time I came to the department in the 1960s. Courtesy of the University of Minnesota Department of Surgery.

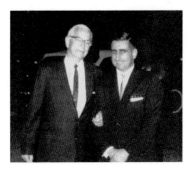

With Owen Wangensteen in the 1970s.

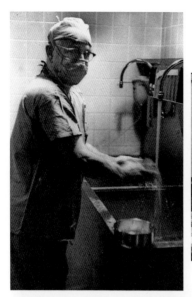
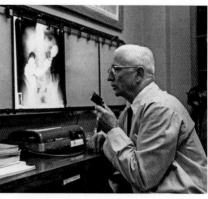
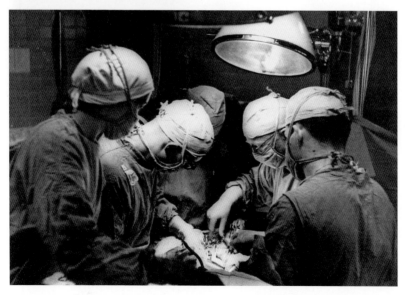

Owen Wangensteen prepping for surgery, in surgery, and reviewing X-rays in the 1960s. Courtesy of the University of Minnesota Department of Surgery.

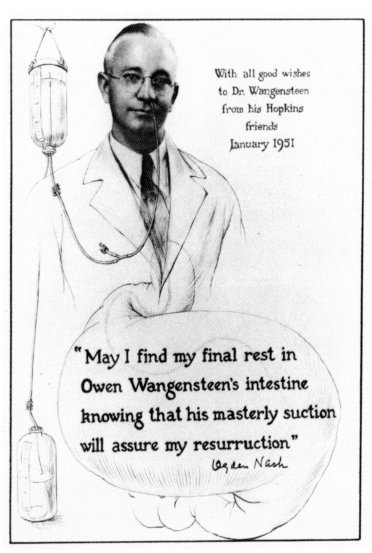

With all good wishes
to Dr. Wangensteen
from his Hopkins
friends
January 1951

"May I find my final rest in
Owen Wangensteen's intestine
knowing that his masterly suction
will assure my resurruction"

Ogden Nash

Wangensteen with his famous suction device, with poem by Ogden Nash. Courtesy of the Wangensteen Historical Library, University of Minnesota.

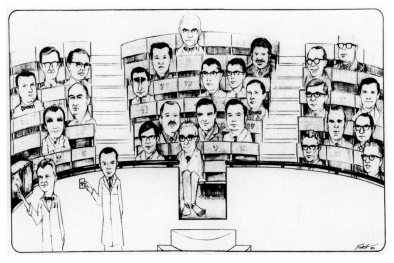

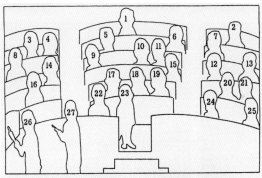

1. Owen H. Wangensteen
2. Victor A. Gilbertson
3. Robert B. Gilsdorf
4. Yoshio Sako
5. Ernesto B. Eusebio
6. Cassius M. C. Ellis
7. Donald G. McQuarrie
8. John B. Lundseth
9. Henry Buchwald
10. Henry A. Sosin
11. Gary W. Lyons
12. Albert W. Sullivan
13. Robert L. Goodale
14. Edward W. Humphrey
15. Arnold S. Leonard
16. Richard C. Lillehei
17. M. Michael Eisenberg
18. Richard L. Varco
19. Demetre M. Nicoloff
20. John S. Najarian
21. Richard L. Simmons
22. Charles F. McKhann
23. William C. Bernstein
24. Aldo R. Castaneda
25. Theodor B. Grage
26. Kurt Amplatz
27. John P. Delaney

The Wangensteen era, circa 1965. Courtesy of the University of Minnesota Department of Surgery.

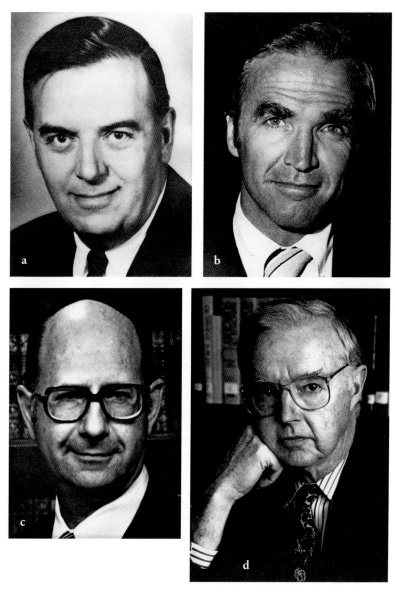

(a) Richard L. Varco; (b) Richard C. Lillehei; (c) Jack Bloch; and (d) John P. Delaney. Courtesy of the University of Minnesota Department of Surgery.

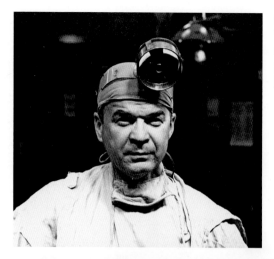

C. Walton Lillehei, the "father of open-heart surgery." Courtesy of the University of Minnesota Archives.

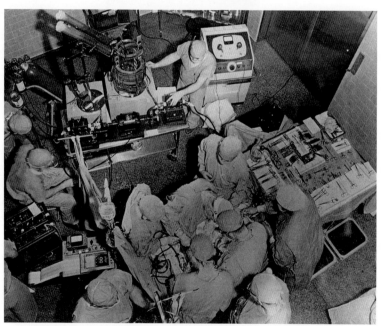

Early open-heart surgery, using the first bubble oxygenator, University of Minnesota. Courtesy of the University of Minnesota Archives.

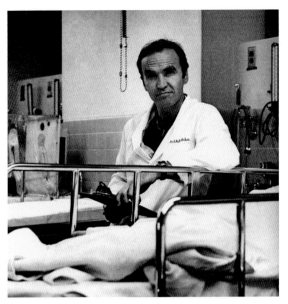

Richard Lillehei at bedside. Courtesy of the University of Minnesota Department of Surgery.

Walton Lillehei and Richard Varco dissecting in the early 1950s. Courtesy of the University of Minnesota Archives.

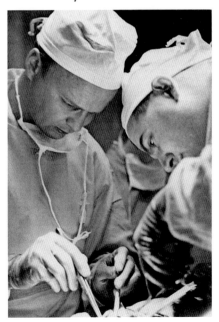

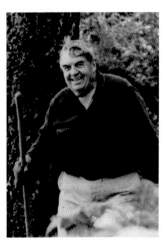

Richard Varco in retirement.

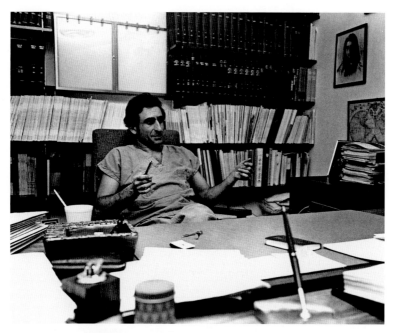

In my office on campus. Courtesy of the University of Minnesota
Archives.

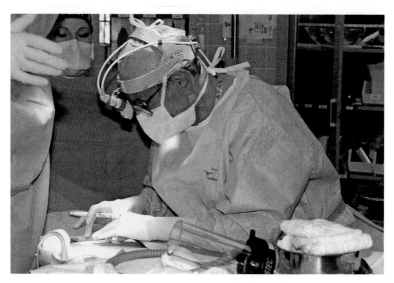

In the operating room. Courtesy of the University of Minnesota Department of Surgery.

Sledding with Jane, Amy, and Claire near our home.

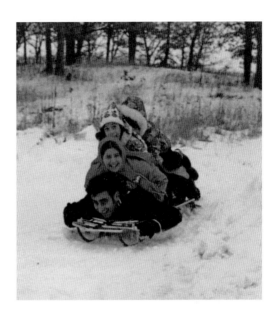

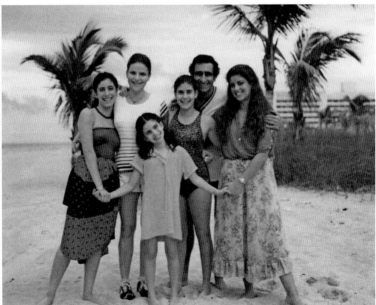

At the beach with Amy, Daisy, Dana, Claire, and Jane.

his eyebrows rose, his eyes twinkled, and he interjected, "A bad fellow." When I related my response to Katz and the silence that followed, his look seemed to say, "I wish I had been there." When I told him about the *Los Angeles Times* article and headline, he chuckled. When I finished my narrative, "The Chief" said, "You bettered Louis Katz. He will not forget or forgive you. You have made a lasting enemy." He paused, and then said, "Show me the man who has no enemies and I will show you the man who has done nothing." He got up, smiled, looked at his watch, and concluded our talk by saying, "The Surgical Forum starts at 8 a.m. You must hurry to the convention center. You don't want to miss any of the papers." In essence, he implied that I had done well in my initiation into academic discourse, and that I should now get on with my life and my work. Our generation of surgeons did not hug. I did not expect a hug or even a pat on the back, and I received none. In our environment, acceptance came through survival. Respect needed to be earned by trial; affection, if it was felt, remained unspoken. I have never forgotten that brief meeting in the lobby of the Fairmont or Dr. Wangensteen's insightful words.

Alongside my laboratory work, I attended classes at the University of Minnesota in biochemistry, physiology, physical chemistry, and statistics. I had never studied statistics in college or in medical school, and an excellent course with Professor Vernon Weckwerth proved essential to my research career.

I did not moonlight in the emergency rooms or on overnight call in other hospitals as many of my peers chose to do. In later years, fewer residents in the surgery department laboratories enrolled for an advanced degree. They spent more time moonlighting than doing research. Some of them earned a good income by this diversion from a full-time research and academic opportunity. Had Dr. Wangensteen found out that a resident was moonlighting, he probably would have discharged him from the program.

For a short period, I did one small bit of extracurricular work to earn extra funds, performing insurance physicals for Lutheran Brotherhood, a fraternal insurance company. I took histories, performed physicals, and submitted urine samples by going to the houses of insurance applicants on my way home, yet never having to spend nights away from home. After several months of performing these examinations, I received a telephone call one evening from the medical director of Lutheran Brotherhood. He informed me that I would no longer be asked to do exams for the company. I inquired why; had I not performed my job well? He said that though I had done well, he had found out I was not Lutheran. I told him that I had never claimed to be Lutheran and asked him what one's religion had to do with performing insurance physicals. He said that hiring only Lutherans was company policy. I hung up. I made no public remonstration, for I certainly did not want Dr. Wangensteen, who probably was Lutheran, to find out that I had been moonlighting, even a little. Because of the long history of Lutheran anti-Semitism, going back to Luther himself, I have always wondered whether I would have been fired by Lutheran Brotherhood had I been Episcopalian or Baptist.

In order to be a degree candidate, I needed to be registered as a graduate student at the University of Minnesota. The tuition for graduate school was not paid for by the Department of Surgery. I was surprised when my fee statement was for an out-of-state student, a sum four times the amount for a Minnesota citizen. I told the board that decided who was and who was not a Minnesota citizen that I lived in Minnesota, that my cars were registered in Minnesota, that I had a Minnesota driver's license, and that I had no residency status in either New York or Nebraska. The board granted me Minnesota citizenship and in-state tuition. I was now an official Minnesotan.

As I entered my laboratory years, I applied for and received financial support for my own income and for my laboratory work. After a series of interviews, I was granted a Helen Hay Whitney Fellowship. The Whitney Foundation is a private charitable trust that competitively selects two to three postdoctoral trainees annually for a two-year fellowship award. These individuals are usually PhD candidates working in the basic sciences. I was one of the few MDs ever chosen by the selection committee. This two-year grant replaced my departmental stipend completely, was paid through the department, and gave me an income somewhat higher than the salaries of third- and fourth-year surgical residents. In addition, the foundation gave a small contribution for academic expenses, such as travel and books.

Before I completed my laboratory years, I applied for an AHA Established Investigator Award. For my final interview, I traveled to Boston to meet with Dean Richard S. Bear of Boston University. He asked me to outline my laboratory accomplishments and future plans. Somewhere in my narrative, I saw that I had lost his attention and that he looked puzzled. I stopped speaking. He stared at me in disbelief and asked if we really had an electron microscope in Minnesota, a tool I would need to do some of the future work I was describing to him. I assured him that we did, and I resisted adding that we had brought it over the prairie in a horse-drawn covered wagon. I later learned from Richard Varco and Walt Lillehei that Katz was doing everything in his power to prevent my receiving this prestigious award, an award rarely given to an MD with clinical practice intentions. I must have had friends somewhere, or my work must have spoken for itself, because I was made an AHA Established Investigator for the next five years, from 1964 to 1969. In receiving this investigatorship, I became independent of departmental state funds and received, via the department, an income that, once again, exceeded the traditional salaries of senior and chief residents. When I completed my residency, Dr. Wangensteen, and later Dr. John Najarian, arranged with the AHA that I could receive additional private practice income without relinquishing my investigatorship.

In 1963, I received my first research grants in what would be a long chain of laboratory funding lasting more than forty-five years. I was awarded a grant from the Life Insurance Medical Research Fund; a grant from the AHA, independent of my investigatorship; and the first in a series of NIH (U.S. Public Health Service) laboratory grants that, over the years, eventually totaled about $100 million. I was happy to inform Dr. Wangensteen that I would not require a second year of departmental laboratory support.

In less than two years at the University of Minnesota, I had secured my own income and laboratory support. With the grant overheads paid directly to the university, I was giving money to, rather than taking money from, the university, which I was able to do for the next fifty years.

⁕ 10 ⁕

Laboratory Funded

*Somewhere, something incredible is
waiting to be known.*

ATTRIBUTED TO CARL SAGAN

With the advent of laboratory funding, I was able to secure laboratory help, including laboratory fellows. Research productivity is enhanced by the addition of personnel, allowing for more work to be performed in a shorter time span by the division of mundane but necessary tasks. Of course, the preferred coworkers are bright, productive, and dedicated. A head of the laboratory or a technician who facilitates procedures and adds new thoughts and concepts becomes a research partner. A well-functioning laboratory is a family of people who like each other, take pleasure in working together, and share in the joy of discovery.

I always incorporated my laboratory fellows into my ongoing projects, but I also encouraged them to have a related project of their own with the full cooperation of the laboratory personnel and the use of our facilities, and at times specialized equipment (e.g., electron microscope) I obtained permission for them to use. I taught them; I learned from them. We often formed enduring relationships. I took great interest in their subsequent, often highly distinguished careers.

My first laboratory technician and head of the laboratory was

Josephine Bertish, an Austrian Jewish Holocaust refugee. She was able to learn, as were both of her successors, to do everything, from complex chemical extractions and radioactivity isotope analyses to animal feed preparation, bleeding, care, and surgical assistance. Josie was a wonderful person who soon became a family friend. She gave us beautiful miniatures painted by her uncle that still hang in our house today. Unfortunately, Josie contracted pancreatic cancer during her tenure in the laboratory and died in her sixties.

I next hired Laurie Fitch, a young woman who worked well with Josie and was an extremely industrious laboratory assistant. Later, Laurie took courses in statistics and trial management and became an indispensable team member of the Coordinating Center of the $65 million Program on the Surgical Control of the Hyperlipidemias (POSCH) grant we received in the 1970s.

My first laboratory fellow was Roger Gebhard, at the time a medical student. He and I worked well together on the laboratory projects that followed my initial experiments. Roger was extremely bright. He chose to enter the specialty of internal medicine and accepted a position at the Veterans Affairs (VA) hospital, where he remained on the faculty in gastroenterology until his retirement. I wanted to continue to work with Roger. I admired his capabilities and his thinking, and I liked him very much. I offered him a partnership in my growing and now well-funded laboratory. However, in his early career, he elected to follow a different path. Many years later, we began to appear on programs together, and we resumed our relationship.

My next laboratory fellow, Marshall Schwartz, became one of my closest lifelong friends. Marshall was a medical student when he started in the laboratory. He was extremely self-possessed, imbued with great self-confidence. He immediately wanted to be responsible for an independent experiment rather than work on ongoing projects. Because his interest was in pediatric surgery, I gave him the opportunity to plan and execute a study in juvenile animals on the efficacy of partial ileal bypass. He did this project exceptionally well, in addition to working with the rest of us. Marshall entered our residency program after medical school and performed superbly. Even Richard Varco thought highly of him and, therefore, incessantly abused him.

Marshall completed his pediatric surgery training in Boston. He became chief of pediatric surgery at the University of Texas, Galveston, and at the University of California, Davis; subsequently, surgeon-in-chief at the Children's Medical Center in Washington, D.C., and professor of surgery and pediatrics and vice chair at Drexel University, and professor at Temple University. He currently holds the title of professor at the Institute for Regenerative Medicine at the Wake Forest School of Medicine. In his illustrious career, he has served as chairman of the Pediatric Surgery Board, president of the American Pediatric Surgical Association, and a nine-year term as a regent of the American College of Surgeons.

Another student in my laboratory's early existence, Peter Agre, was the son of two University of Minnesota professors. He was an eager learner with an unquenchable curiosity. He was well liked and fit in nicely with our nascent laboratory group. Peter went on to obtain his MD degree and made his career at Johns Hopkins, not primarily in clinical medicine but in basic research. In 2003, he was awarded the Nobel Prize in chemistry for his work in the elucidation of the rapid transfer tubules in cell membranes.

In addition to my first experiments, a great deal of work was accomplished during these two years of dedicated research time. By blood cholesterol-4-$C14$ analyses, I, and later with coworkers, defined the sites for cholesterol absorption after oral feeding of a test dose in rabbits with various segments of their small intestine bypassed. We demonstrated that cholesterol can be absorbed in the entire small intestine but is preferentially absorbed in the ileum, the farthest segment of small intestine. We showed that bile salt absorption was also primarily localized to the terminal ileum. This work was essential confirmation of the physiologic basis for the results of the partial ileal bypass operation, and that ileal bowel diversion from the intestinal stream will result in lowering the blood cholesterol concentration. I also confirmed in human partial ileal bypass patients that vitamin B12 is primarily absorbed in the ileum, attesting to the necessity for partial ileal bypass patients to require vitamin B12 supplementation.

I showed in rabbits that atherosclerosis and myocardial infarctions (documented by electrocardiograms, transient cardiac arrest arteriograms, and tissue pathology) can be induced solely by a hypercholesterolemia diet. I showed that partial ileal bypass in rabbits would prevent atherosclerosis and myocardial infarctions and actually reverse established atherosclerotic lesions. In addition, performing electrocardiograms and arteriograms in rabbits, as well as inducing myocardial infarctions in rabbits, were original and novel contributions to the research methodology of the time. Several years later, we presented our partial ileal bypass results at the American College of Surgeons with a far better reception than the one received from Dr. Katz at the American Heart Association. All of our work was accepted for publication in prestigious journals.

The cholesterol/atherosclerosis hypothesis states that high cholesterol levels will induce atherosclerosis and its sequelae; the hypothesis derivative converse statement is that lowering cholesterol levels will retard or even reverse atherosclerosis. Our data proved both the primary and the converse statements—in essence, changing the cholesterol/atherosclerosis hypothesis into a fact.

I maintained my functioning laboratory for nearly fifty years. On returning to the clinical services in 1964, in addition to my full clinical responsibilities I continued to run my laboratory. Over the years, our work gained recognition and was amply funded by the NIH and other organizations.

During these laboratory years, I started a working relationship with Dr. Richard Moore. Dick Moore was a postdoctoral (MD) student with several years of internal medicine training working in Dr. Frantz's laboratory on cholesterol and bile acid metabolism. He was extremely intelligent, as well as meticulous. He did not take shortcuts. He was precise, and his research results could be trusted. He worked slowly and carefully, except once, when a blender containing rabbit feces in preparation for quantitative stool analysis exploded and coated Dr. Frantz's laboratory with a fine patina of poop.

Over the years, Dick and I were coauthors of twenty-six papers. Our joint efforts demonstrated the effects of partial ileal bypass on increasing body cholesterol synthesis to compensate for the increased fecal excretion of cholesterol, as cholesterol and as the foundation of bile acids; cholesterol turnover; and the plasma concentration where eventually the body's cholesterol pools stabilized. The body's cholesterol pools can be divided into the freely miscible (blood, liver) and the less freely miscible (body organs and tissues). The latter includes the arteries and the formation of cholesterol-rich atherosclerotic plaques. Although the partial ileal bypass increased cholesterol synthesis and turnover, the miscible pools of most mammals (including humans) decreased in content. Thus, not only was the blood cholesterol concentration markedly reduced by the partial ileal bypass, but so was the cholesterol content of the arterial wall.

In these two research years, I completed the course work for my MA in biochemistry and my PhD in surgery. My physiology professor was erratic, absent-minded, and not the best lecturer, but he was a genial man who loved to teach and gave individual attention to his undergraduate and graduate students. Jack Bloch, a sailor, was asked by this teacher for advice on how to build a partially prefabricated sailboat. Jack reviewed the plans and told him the boat would be larger than his garage (his workshop). He also told him that the single mast had to be placed through the boat deck and secured to the keel of the boat. The professor, however, insisted on building the boat in his garage and subsequently had to destroy the front overhang of the garage to get the boat out. Again, not listening to Jack's advice, he anchored the mast to the deck rather than to the keel. In his first sail, with a good puff of wind, the mast fell, ripping out most of the deck. This incident typified so many of his undertakings that he, though extremely well liked, was a source of great head-shaking in the medical school. Because of this reputation, when he invented a cardiotonic drug, the university refused to patent it, and he did so on his own. He made several million dollars, and I was very happy for him.

In contrast to this well-liked teacher, we were taught by a physiologist who was arrogant, condescending, rude, and a mediocre teacher into the bargain. One day, he was speeding north on Interstate 35W when he was stopped by a Minneapolis police car. He shouted at the officers that he had to get to the operating room at the University of Minnesota for an emergency case. He was a PhD, not an MD, and certainly not a surgeon. The officers told him to follow them, and, with siren blasting and lights flashing, they headed down 35W toward the university. The physiologist followed them for a short distance and then suddenly turned off. The police made a U-turn against traffic, chased and cornered him and demanded an explanation. He replied that he thought he was taking a shortcut. The police officers, now becoming suspicious, told him to follow them and not to deviate from their course again. When they arrived in front of the hospital, the man leaped out of his car, thanked the police officers, entered the building, and ran up the flight of stairs to the operating rooms. Instead of leaving, the officers accompanied him. As he entered the operating room suite, he shouted, "Where is my patient? Where is my patient?" The head of the operating rooms, a seasoned and crusty old chief nurse, looked up from the control desk and asked, "Who are you?" The police officers questioned the head nurse, who said she had never seen the man before. They put him in handcuffs and took him to jail. Only a day later, after the university had paid a fine and the dean had personally vouched for him, was he released.

For some reason, my favorite studies in biochemistry, which included lipid chemistry with Ivan Frantz, required that I take a semester of physical chemistry. Jack Bloch had the same requirement, and we took the course together. The instructor was younger than we were and very rigid in his requirements. The first half of this one-point course consisted of learning the principles of analysis of chemical phenomena by physics concepts, essentially the art of applied mathematics. The second half consisted of problem solving and soon came down to calculating the surface tension of a soap bubble as it expanded. Week after week, we expanded this virtual soap bubble and were scheduled to do so for the remainder of the course. Jack and I had learned what we wanted to learn, had passed all the quizzes, and had earned A's in our midterm examination. We suggested to the instructor that we stop coming to class to expand the soap bubble, that we not take the final exam, and that he give us a pass grade, because that was all we needed for our graduate-school requirements. The instructor threw a fit, threatened our graduate-school standing, and refused our request. Jack and I continued to calculate the expansion of this damn soap bubble, took the final examination, and received, as I recall, A's for the course. The instructor had no choice but to grade us free of his subjective resentment toward us. He who lives by numbers must grade by numbers.

My favorite recollection of postgraduate schooling was taking the simplified French course for PhD candidates at the same time as Daisy. She needed to demonstrate proficiency in two languages for her PhD in English literature. At that time, all PhD candidates, even PhD candidates in the sciences, had to fulfill the same language requirement. We both tested out of German, Daisy quite easily, for she could read and write German. I had somewhat more difficulty. I speak German fluently, but I was, and remain, a German illiterate. I took the examination sheet and sounded the words out for myself, because by sight the words were meaningless to me. The test monitor told me to stop mumbling; I told him that I had to mumble to "read." He exiled me to a corner of the room. I mumbled my way through the test and passed. For my second language, I signed up for Latin. Daisy, who had some Latin and Greek in her schooling, would educate and concurrently irritate me by dissecting English words into their Latin roots. I wanted to be able to do this as well, especially with respect to medical terminology. To my surprise, I was told by the graduate school that Latin was not an approved medical language for a PhD in surgery. This was perhaps my first realization that the administrative policies of the University of Minnesota were not necessarily based on rational decisions. I selected French, and Daisy and I signed up for the same course.

This was a very busy time for me in the laboratory, and I rarely, if ever, worked on my French outside the classroom. Not so Daisy; she was fairly proficient in the language and increased her proficiency by her application to the subject. There was only one exam—the final —for determination of the pass or fail grade. The night before the final examination, I studied and memorized the requisite vocabulary. Daisy and I took the exam, and on the way home we discussed it. We agreed that I had translated the vocabulary list correctly. My paragraph translation from French to English was not as accurate. Our conversation went something like this:

ME: There was a king *(roi)*, who had three daughters *(trois filles)*; they lived in a château on the Loire.

DAISY: So far so good.

ME: One day, strange men came over the mountains.

DAISY: There were no mountains, but yes, strange men came.

ME: I lost a lot in the middle, however, because these stories usually end with a "forever after," and I believe the king died *(mort)*. I wrote that the strange men married the three daughters, the king lived to a ripe old age before he died, and the couples lived happily ever after in the château on the Loire.

DAISY: Not quite. The strangers, who did not come over any mountains, invaded and pillaged the land, killed the king, which was why he was *"mort,"* raped the three daughters, burned the château, and left.

ME: This is not good.

DAISY: No. It is not.

The day that grades were posted in the classroom building, I checked on the results. I read, "Emilie Buchwald, pass. Henry Buchwald, pass." I was amazed, and, because I was not a young student who would have left well enough alone, I went to see our French instructor. Unlike my physical chemistry teacher, this man was mature and welcomed me to his office with a smile. I asked him, "How could you pass me?" He responded, "I could not very well pass your wife and not you. And I have rarely laughed so hard on reading any translation." We both laughed and that was that. Daisy and I had each fulfilled our PhD language requirements.

Because I was on call every other night and weekend, and we lived in an isolated cul-de-sac, I wanted a guard dog to protect my family. In the spring of 1962, we acquired our German shepherd, Buck, from two sisters who lived in a rural location and bred large shepherd dogs with pedigreed stock from Germany. Buck was a beautiful dog who grew to about one hundred pounds. We realized in retrospect that we did a very poor job of socializing Buck as a puppy. No one told us how important it was to introduce him to many different people. The result was that he was totally dedicated to the family but hostile to anyone else, including policemen, mailmen, all strangers, and even visitors, at least until we convinced him simply to be aloof rather than antagonistic.

Buck and our daughter Amy were "puppies" together. They would sit next to each other and bark in unison. Two-year-old Amy shared her food with Buck and occasionally fed him toothpaste. If she wanted to keep an object safe—a ball, for example—she would open his massive jaws and place the ball inside. One day, I took Amy and Buck with me in the back of our station wagon to buy a newspaper and some milk. When I reached the store, Amy was asleep. I decided to leave the two of them in the car, and opened the back window a couple of inches for ventilation. I was in the store only a few minutes when I came out to find a crowd around the back of the car, shouting for someone to get the police. One industrious stranger was thrusting an umbrella back and forth through the slightly open window. I rushed to the car to find Buck protecting Amy from this mob of well-intentioned busybodies who seemed to believe the dog was endangering the child. Buck's hackles were up, his huge teeth were bared, and he had just crunched the umbrella being thrust at him. One of his gigantic front paws was protecting the sleeping Amy. As I rushed to disperse the crowd, Buck was lunging at the window. I quieted the crowd; I quieted Buck; Amy slept on.

Just as exciting and memorable was a winter night at bedtime. Buck was out on the screened front porch in the insulated doghouse I had built for him, where he spent his nights. We were turning off lights when we realized that Amy was missing. Daisy, Jane, and I frantically searched the house. Amy was not to be found. It was below zero outside. We realized that if Amy had gone out, Buck would have given the alarm or stayed with her. When we went out to the porch, we found Buck and Amy cuddled up together in the doghouse. Amy explained that she wanted to be sure that "Bucky" was all right in the cold. We reassured her that he was and brought her back into the house.

In the summer of 1962, the Blochs—Jack, Gretchen, and their oldest son, Robbie—and the four Buchwalds rented a cabin for a long weekend in northern Minnesota. We had a wonderful time walking forest trails, cooking dinners, and watching Buck cavort in the woods. Gretchen and Daisy were both pregnant. A few days after our return, they both sustained miscarriages. We blamed this odd coincidence on something in the water, or on some other unknown cause related to our northern trip. All of us were depressed about this double misery. Gretchen soon became pregnant again, and nine months later delivered the Blochs's second son, Paul.

Daisy became pregnant again in December 1963, and all went well until September 1964. She was two weeks past her due date when labor pains began. She was hospitalized on the evening of September 16, 1964. By the time I arrived at the hospital the next morning, having seen Jane off to school and Amy to our babysitter, the medical student who had been assigned to listen to the fetal heart sounds reported no audible heartbeat. Daisy said, quite desperately, that she felt movement, and she asked Konnie Prem to perform an emergency cesarean section. He performed the surgery, but the baby was dead. Prem had no explanation. The pathologist was vague and actually uncomfortable about having no specific diagnosis. Our baby boy, apparently normal and without any congenital defects, had, we believed, died needlessly. Daisy and I were in shock. As I write this memoir in my eighties, I remember the death of this child as if it happened yesterday.

I returned home that evening to explain to Jane, age six, and Amy, age three, why they would not have a brother coming home with Mom, and that Mom would have to remain in the hospital for several days. They cried. I wanted to cry with them, but that was not my role. Then an extraordinary thing happened. We noticed a small bird, a sparrow, I believe, flying around inside our house, crashing into walls, desperate in its panic. How it got in I will never know. It was strange, unexplained. I caught the bird and held it gently in my hands. I took the children with me to the door. I said to them that the bird was the spirit of their brother, asking our permission to let him fly to heaven. I opened the door and let the bird fly free. We wished him well on his journey.

✢ 11 ✢

Senior Resident

The most universal quality is diversity.
_____

MICHEL DE MONTAIGNE,
"Of the Resemblance of Children to
Their Fathers," *Essays*, 1580

I returned to the clinical services in March 1964. By the end of
June, I had completed the four months I owed for my third clinical year of postmedical-school training. July began my fourth year
of residency, today referred to as the senior residency year. The fifth
and final year of clinical training would be the chief residency.

For my first clinical rotation, from March through June 1964, I
was once again on Purple Surgery with Dr. Wangensteen, who was
pleased by the early positive clinical results with the partial ileal
bypass. The chief resident for this rotation on Purple Surgery was
Ward O. Griffen Jr., a fabulous surgeon and mentor who became
a lifelong friend. Even after the Griffens and their seven children
moved to Lexington, Kentucky, where Ward served as chief of
surgery, and later when he moved to Philadelphia as the chair of
the American Board of Surgery, our families maintained contact.
During this 1964 rotation with Ward, I greatly increased my operative skills and clinical judgment.

In July, I started my senior year of residency with four months
on Blue Surgery. The chief of Blue Surgery was John Perry, an excel-

lent surgeon and teacher, as well as an extremely nice person. As I mentioned earlier, John had a discernible tremor in both hands until they or the instruments they held touched an operative surface. Then his tremor totally disappeared.

A Texan by birth, accent, and bearing, John announced in 1964 that he had accepted a job offer in Texas and would be leaving immediately. He was well liked, and we organized a staff/resident party at Charlie's Café Exceptionale, then the best and most elegant restaurant in Minneapolis. As a farewell gift, we gave him an expensive set of luggage. Several weeks after the party, John said he had changed his mind and would instead become chief of surgery at Ramsey County Medical Center (now Regions Hospital) in St. Paul. We demanded, partly in jest, that he return his travel luggage, which he did not do. His career at Ramsey County brought that institution up several rungs in excellence and prestige. It also cemented an academic relationship with them for a residency rotation with our department.

In November, I moved on to Red Surgery. Alan Thal had accepted a job in Detroit, and Rich Lillehei was now head of the service. Rich was brilliant and mercurial, a gastrointestinal and cardiac surgeon who, as stated earlier, performed the world's first pancreas transplant at Minnesota. He taught me that when a patient of ours came in with a problem requiring hospitalization, I was to admit that patient to our surgical service and only then request the appropriate consultative help. Thus, though we admitted individuals with primary cardiac, gynecologic, otolaryngologic, and dermatologic concerns, among many others, we acted as their primary physicians and coordinated their care.

In later years, I found this practice very useful because the Department of Medicine's official policy was that when an internist's long-standing patient was admitted to the hospital—even though he had taken care of that patient for years—he would no longer be in charge and the patient would fall instead under the management of the internist who was on the monthlong rotation on the medical unit in the hospital. Further, an acute medical admission would be seen first by a medical student, then by an intern, then by the resident, and, only at a conference or at rounds the next day, by the attending physician. These rules virtually guaranteed that the primary physician lost all control over ongoing patient care, and that patient care responsibility started at the bottom rather than at the top of the clinical ladder of knowledge and experience. This system seemed, and seems, nonsensical to me. Once I became an attending surgeon, I adopted Rich Lillehei's practice of admitting all acute patients of mine, or those referred to me, to my service, regardless of their main problem. In particular, I admitted the patients of Dr. Naip Tuna, the best cardiologist at the university, and gave him a free hand in my patient order book, a privilege he did not enjoy on the inpatient service of his own department.

On a regular basis, Rich would argue with his older brother Walt about patients, concepts, and, most frequently, privileges. One day the two Lilleheis were standing in the hall in front of the operating room control desk having a long, vociferous debate about who was entitled to the 7 a.m. start in a shared operating room the following morning. As they were shouting and gesticulating, Allen Moberg, a resident at the time, put a hand on each of their shoulders and said, "Boys, why don't you take it home to mother?" Irreverence, as a rule, increases from generation to generation; however, during my nearly sixty-year tenure in the University of Minnesota Department of Surgery, decorum and permissible behavior have gone in the opposite direction. Departmental interactions have certainly become more polite, but often more regimented. I do not believe this is a change for the better. On the contrary, in my opinion, it is detrimental to academic freedom of discourse.

Rich was a people person and generous. He and his wife, BJ,

invited residents to their home, located near Lake of the Isles in Minneapolis, on a regular basis. They served superb food, excellent drinks, and provided amiable argumentation. Rich also invited residents out for dinner and entertainment at meeting venues of the American College of Surgeons and the American Heart Association, especially if the meetings were in New Orleans or San Francisco. Bourbon Street in New Orleans offered strip shows, bars, and, in particular, the original jazz classics played by the old-timers of the Preservation Hall Jazz Band in a storefront room for dollars tossed into a hat. Broadway in San Francisco also offered banjo bands, the players often seated on a platform behind the bar. These banjo joints were Rich's favorite haunts. Many of the players knew him, and, when they did not, he introduced himself. He was invited, or he invited himself, to go to the platform and sit in on the drums. He could, and would, stay long into the night at this activity. Rich was not an introvert.

I remember one particular trip with Rich. We were in Philadelphia for the annual meeting of the Society of University Surgeons. It was 1968, the year of my election to fellowship into the group. We were at the Barclay Hotel, which in its day was the most exclusive hotel in the city. Rich invited me to breakfast with Joseph E. Murray from Harvard, later awarded the Nobel Prize in medicine for performing the first kidney transplant between identical twins. The dining room was ornate; place settings were of the best porcelain and silverware; waitstaff, who outnumbered the guests, were at attention beside polished sideboards displaying coffee and tea services. When we sat down, Rich and Dr. Murray were immediately deep in conversation. Rich told me to order whatever I wanted. I perused the menu. All dishes were exorbitantly expensive; each item was à la carte, including coffee, toast, and an order of jams and marmalade. None of the waitstaff came over after we were seated.

Rich, accustomed to Midwestern mores where the breakfast client is cheerily greeted by the waiter or waitress and immediately offered coffee, kept gesturing to the waiters. He got no response. "What the hell," he said, got up, went to the sideboard, picked up a pot of coffee, and walked back to our table. Now waiters converged on our table, insisted on pouring the coffee, and one finally took our order. I mentioned to Rich that everything was extremely expensive. He waved off my hesitation. The three of us ordered eggs and breakfast meats. Neither he nor Dr. Murray consulted the menu. Again, time went by and no food came. We had a meeting to attend, and we were hungry. Next to us sat a meticulously dressed elderly man. He was alone, reading the *Philadelphia Inquirer* section by section, turning the pages carefully and folding them into long vertical columns. He had ordered the à la carte toast served on its special silver salver, and the à la carte jams and marmalades, each on individual platters. Rich assumed that these items came with the breakfast order and were not "extras." Plainly, the gentleman at the other table was through with them. Rich got up and walked over to his table, smiled, picked up the salvers of toast and spreads and returned to our table. The gentleman looked outraged. He signed his bill, folded up his paper, and, casting a disgusted look at us, walked out. I told Rich what had just happened and why. Rich laughed and said, "He'll get over it."

Rich was original, a free spirit, stubborn, and an athlete. I was on call one night when a howling blizzard closed all city streets. By dawn, cars parked outdoors were snowy humps, snow-packed streets were clogged, and the city snowplows were making little headway. Schools and the university were closed; city services were suspended. The city was white, cold, and quiet. Very few if any went to work that day, except for Rich, who had surgery to perform and patients to see, and who would not accept being dictated to by the

weather. Rich put on his cross-country skis and skied the five miles
to work. His photograph, on his skis, was in the paper the next day.

On another occasion, in early winter before the frozen city lakes
were designated safe for ice skating, Rich went skating around Lake
of the Isles, ignoring the "Ice Unsafe" signs. A patrol car driving the
lake perimeter pulled alongside him and the officer ordered Rich
to come off the ice. Rich responded that skating on the lake was his
concern and his risk and not the concern of the police. He skated
away. Other patrol cars were radioed to the lake; police officers on
foot ran along the lake edge. Rich eluded them for some time by
speeding away and skating farther out on the unsafe ice. Finally, he
surrendered, was arrested, and once again had his photograph in
the paper. He maintained his reputation as a public idol.

I had one unpleasant episode with Rich Lillehei during this
rotation on Red Surgery. One night when I was on call and had
completed all the necessary work and checked on all my patients,
I went over to my laboratory and worked there on calculations for
an hour. When I returned to the main hospital, I was being frantically paged; there were no electronic pagers or cell phones in the
1960s. It was Rich, asking about an emergency patient being admitted. He asked where I had been. I told him. He admonished me;
more than that, he castigated me for dereliction of my primary
responsibility to the surgical service. He was right. I was wrong.
One apologizes in situations such as this, but that apology is quite
meaningless. Acknowledging my mistake was what was necessary. I
did that, and the matter was closed. I do not know if Rich remembered this event, but I have never forgotten it.

I spent the final four months of senior residency on White Surgery. The leadership of the service had not changed. The head of
White was still Joe Aust; the other senior staff were Ted Grage and
Al Sullivan. Aust and Grage operated often and had difficult, fascinating cases.

This time period was the most amiable one for my relationship with Joe Aust. We played tennis together almost every Sunday. We were evenly matched and did not tire of the competition. I had taken up tennis in medical school when I realized I would never again find twenty-one other people to play soccer with, and I had tired of swimming laps in a swimming pool. Furthermore, tennis courts were far more available than swimming pools. Running had not yet become a national hobby.

I believe it was Ted who introduced me to the Haskells, who owned the best liquor store in Minneapolis. Bennie Haskell, a former boxer, bootlegger, and felon, was forbidden by law to wait on customers. He sat in the back of the store with clients, drinking samples of the best European vintage wines. His wife, Fritzi Haskell, served favored long-term customers, keeping a book of the choices and brands of liquors preferred by some of the leading citizens of the Twin Cities. Ted liked wine, good beers, and various high-alcohol beverages.

During this rotation, my friendship with Al Sullivan deepened. He was a scholar and a reader who prided himself on his ability to speak fluent French. He did not seek to do large resections like many academic surgeons of that time. He contented himself with utilitarian procedures, hernias and gallbladders, performed cleanly and meticulously. He loved to lecture and was without doubt the best didactic teacher of medical students in our department. Years later, when I was a full professor, I argued with John Najarian, then chairman of the Department of Surgery, for Al's promotion to full professor. Najarian stated that Al Sullivan did not perform "big" surgery and had no research credits. I countered that as a department we were charged with the task of teaching students in the medical school, a pursuit that gave us our academic titles, and that Al was our best teacher of medical students.

Al died relatively young of a brain tumor. He never lost his intellectual curiosity, his sense of equanimity, or his dignity. My last visit with him was at his home in St. Paul. We sat in the living room and he analyzed what he found to be an interesting phenomenon: the spreading brain tumor was beginning to rob him of his formidable English vocabulary, although his command of French remained intact. He was a fine person with a rare sense of decency.

🔸 12 🔸

Colleagues

The greatest gift of life is friendship,
and I have received it.

HUBERT H. HUMPHREY,
in Carl Solberg, *Hubert Humphrey:*
A Biography, 1984

My fellow residents as well as the faculty shaped the legacy of the Wangensteen era. The stories of some who became my friends and colleagues over the years are well worth relating.

Of course, there was Dr. Jack Bloch; he and his family appear throughout this narrative.

My close friend of fifty-plus years, Dr. John (Jack) P. Delaney, completed his undergraduate schooling at Notre Dame and his medical school and internship at the University of Minnesota. Like most residents in my time, Jack fulfilled a two-year obligation in the armed services. He was stationed in Korea in an army unit called the Korean Military Advisory Group. Military experience matured us all and made us less susceptible to the inherent infantilizing of a training program at many academic institutions. Jack exhibited this maturity in his reasoning, his actions, and his solid independence. He never acted precipitously; he did not engage in frivolous encounters; he made his decisions based on his own logical thinking and his unshakable sense of right and wrong. He was a pillar of integrity, trusted for his word and deeds.

During our residency years, I was introduced to Jack's unique sense of humor. He was a member of Dr. Wangensteen's laboratory, as were most of the residents selected by Dr. Wangensteen as suitable for future careers in academia. During his laboratory tenure, pure ethyl alcohol bottles went missing, bottles of 100 percent alcohol, which, with a little flavoring (e.g., orange juice), made an excellent party drink.

After some research, Jack found a tasteless vital dye, colorless in alcohol and Kelly green in an acid aqueous media. He placed the dye in one of the ethyl alcohol bottles. The next day, one of the laboratory technicians came in to Jack in a frantic state, saying that his urine was a bright green. Jack calmly told him that this was a most interesting fact, and that he was fired.

Soon after we achieved faculty attending status, Jack and I became clinical partners on Red Surgery. For about forty years, we looked out for each other's interests, mutually promoted department initiatives, and covered patients in seamless fashion. We lived together the critical years of general surgery that gave way to specialization. We worked with six department heads and through four deans.

Throughout our careers, I have avoided sitting on faculty selection committees. Jack, on the other hand, served on many of them, especially those selecting a new dean. I asked him why he wasted his time in this manner. He responded that it was in our interest, as a department, to select the appropriate person to be the dean. He said he always promoted the weakest candidate because a weak dean made it easier to maintain Department of Surgery autonomy, whereas a strong dean was dangerous to that autonomy. I responded that a strong dean could be good for all of the medical school, including our department. "Maybe so," Jack said, "but it would be taking a risk. Even if it proved successful during that dean's tenure, it would set a precedent for a strong dean, which, sooner or later, would be detrimental for us."

At a meeting of the prestigious American Surgical Association, a professor of surgery presented his series of pancreatic sphincter of Oddi operations. The sphincter is, at best, a poorly defined structure, and the surgeon stressed that the operation might need to be repeated two to three times to achieve a pain-free state. Jack rose to his feet during the discussion period and stated, "I have found that if you operate enough times on a patient, he or she will stop complaining."

Jack's independent research laboratory worked on methods to prevent postoperative adhesions, as well as creating nonreactive mesh prostheses for hernia repairs. Several patents have resulted from his work. His laboratory was endowed by a grateful patient, and he maintained an active research facility for many years past his retirement.

During the chairmanship of John Najarian, individual surgical billing was replaced by a unified departmental billing structure that worked relatively well. I had no choice but to join because my personal income from the American Heart Association Established Investigatorship Award had to be funneled through the department. Richard Varco warned against any centralization of billing and its accompanying control of income; however, he was no longer clinically active when this change occurred. Jack held out against considerable pressure and remained independent in his billing. He did so as well when the departmental system was swallowed up by the University of Minnesota Physicians (UMP) billing system, and we, the entire clinical faculty, essentially became employees of a self-serving, fiscal entity. By his stance, Jack lost out on certain retirement benefits but maintained control over his income above his base salary and, most important, his monetary freedom and independence.

This fierce individualism at a university tending more and more toward central authority and a governance system characterized by business-world ethics may have been costly for Jack in other than financial ways. He had established a national reputation in breast surgery and the management of breast cancer. He and Dr. Byrl James (B. J.) Kennedy, a world-renowned oncologist who revolutionized the management of breast cancer, had long dreamed of building a university hospital breast center. They planned it, they designed it, they found university space for it, and they raised more than two million dollars for this enterprise. The university established the Breast Center. It elected, however, to move it across the Mississippi River to our Fairview System partner and, instead of putting Jack and B. J. in charge, it chose a local surgeon with limited experience to head the center. The center soon folded; it would have been the first of its kind dedicated to the care of women afflicted with the most frequent cancer in women.

After the announcement of his retirement, while Jack and I were eating lunch together at a small off-campus Vietnamese restaurant, I asked him why he had made the decision to retire, though he was active and in general good health. He simply answered, "When the crap of the day outweighs the fun, it is time to go." Jack was always wise; he was my mentor on how to live life and make important decisions.

Dr. Robert (Bob) Goodale was another individual I greatly admired—a person of wealth who did not need to work but chose to. As a surgeon, he worked long hours and was devoted to his patients. Although he was a gentle person, when dedicated to a task he pursued it regardless of opposition. He went to Japan to study endoscopy and laparoscopy; in the 1960s, the Japanese were well ahead of us in the clinical initiation of these techniques. Bob was encouraged in these endeavors by Dr. Wangensteen but discouraged by Dr. Wangensteen's successor, Dr. Najarian. Yet he persisted, becoming the first certified practitioner of these skills at the University of Minnesota Hospital. He also mastered rudimentary Japanese during this endeavor. He taught laparoscopy to Jack Delaney and to me, and for a period of time we three represented laparoscopic surgery at the university. We banded together to pressure John Najarian to hire young laparoscopic surgeons, but without success.

In his retirement, Bob traveled with his wife, Kathy, exercised, played the French horn, pursued his Japanese- and French-language proficiency, and in all his endeavors exhibited the natural, quiet dignity of the gentleman he always was.

Dr. Donald (Don) McQuarrie, another resident of independent means, was a superlative surgeon and teacher. As noted earlier, Don and I were together on the Anoka service and during my first rotation on Purple Surgery. When he completed residency, he took a staff position at the VA Hospital and succeeded Dr. Edward Humphrey as the chair of surgery. He was one of the best head and neck surgeons in the Twin Cities, and the VA offered him the opportunity to operate as much or as little as he wished. He did not need to operate to earn his living. It was said that Don would occasionally forget to pick up his VA paycheck.

One of my most outstanding colleagues, Dr. Demetre (Nick) Nicoloff, finished the residency program a couple of years before I did. He went to the VA to hone his gastrointestinal surgery skills. He, too, was a Varco disciple. There was an understanding among Nick, Varco, and myself that Nick would become Varco's gastrointestinal surgeon colleague and I would become the junior cardiovascular surgeon. During my chief residency year, I upset this anticipation by deciding against pursuing cardiovascular surgery and selecting gastrointestinal surgery instead. In the 1960s, during this adolescent period for cardiovascular procedures, cardiovascular surgery required the surgeon to be an intensivist and to spend his nonoperative hours, often into the evening and through the night, in the intensive-care unit, taking care of critical patients. This schedule left little or no time for basic bench research, and I did not intend to give that up. Nick, concurrently and quite independently, decided to be a cardiovascular surgeon instead of specializing in gastrointestinal surgery. He moved back to the university from the VA after Walt Lillehei's departure for Cornell and Richard Varco's operative inactivity and eventual retirement. He became the leading cardiovascular surgeon in our department. We made complementary career changes that worked out well for both of us, and, in a sense, satisfied Varco's intentions for us. During our time together on the faculty, Nick and I often went to the Coffman Union Faculty Club after Saturday morning conference for its juicy hamburgers. We were good friends and regulars at poker parties.

When Nick's reputation as a cardiovascular surgeon was established, he wanted greater recognition and the opportunity to make more money than a university appointment and practice would generate. At the same time, Varco demanded that Nick perform basic research at the expense of his time in the operating room. Naturally enough, they clashed. Nick threatened to leave the university, and Varco threatened to fire him. I interceded. I talked with Nick, who was unsure of what to do. I went to Varco and was told to mind my own business. I went to Najarian, chair of surgery at that time, and asked him to give Nick a clinical surgery title and a promotion; he, too, told me to mind my own business. Nick left the university and started the Twin Cities' major cardiovascular surgery group and cardiac center at Abbott Northwestern Hospital in Minneapolis. Subsequently, I saw Nick only at meetings and dinners of organizations we both belonged to.

A senior colleague who played an important role in our department was Dr. Arnold S. (Arnie) Leonard. He was the first fully trained pediatric surgeon at the university, and broadened his education by specialty training at outside institutions. With his twin brother, a nonuniversity pediatrician, Arnie established the largest pediatric surgery practice in the area. He operated at several hospitals in addition to the university hospital, including Minneapolis's Children's Hospital, St. Paul's Children's Hospital, and Abbott Northwestern Hospital. He commuted swiftly from institution to institution in his car, eating en route. His desire for speed while driving frightened many of the residents traveling with him.

When UMP was formed, Arnie, like Varco, foresaw that in a short time it would become the fiscal entity that ruled clinical practice rather than a helpful fiscal agent for the clinical faculty. Indeed, the physicians who supported the concept of a single university billing agent became the employees of UMP, and instead of the democratic governance that was promised, UMP leadership initiated a bureaucracy of administrators; certain physicians came to dictate the earnings of others, rather than seeing patients themselves. Above all, to support this dysfunctional organization, UMP taxed the billing collections, which were considerably lower than community standards. Rather than submit to UMP, Arnie resigned his academic professorship and secured a clinical professorship, and with it independence from UMP. He knew that as long as he was bringing in research funds and clinical moneys, the Academic Health Center and the university medical school would not revoke his office, laboratory space, or operating privileges, including the services of the surgery department's residents. By this simple exchange of titles, he escaped what the rest of us accepted because of our emotional, perhaps irrational, attachment to an academic title.

Working to understand and influence cancer mechanisms, Arnie's laboratory has been, and continues to be, funded by the traditional public and industry sources, as well as by himself, even well after his retirement. The laboratory is now mentored and led by his successor in pediatric surgery, Dr. Daniel Saltzman. Arnie has for many years been an avid hunter. He purchased a large tract of unzoned land along the banks of the Minnesota River and converted it into a game reserve. During hunting season, he charges hunters to use his property and he publishes a magazine for hunters. He contributes all the proceeds from these ventures to support his laboratory and his laboratory fellows.

When our daughter Amy was twelve, she came home from school with abdominal pain. As it happened, I was home that morning and realized that she had classic appendicitis. I called Arnie and we rushed to the hospital. He had an operating room ready and a staff in attendance. The appendectomy went smoothly, and Amy left the hospital that afternoon. Arnie again came into Amy's life several years later when she was getting married. He grew flowers and prided himself on his dahlias. For the wedding, he took it upon himself to decorate our home with a profusion of beautiful flowers from his garden. Arnie is a generous person, always available to those who come to him for advice or assistance. On retirement, he completed a short history of the University of Minnesota Department of Surgery, citing the accomplishments of our peers and mentors.

✤ 13 ✤

Chief Resident

It is my conviction that great teachers
focus as importantly on the unknown
as the known. Our disciplines advance
solely by pushing back the topography
of ignorance. When the challenge
of the unknown captures the professor's
students, the teacher's mission
is fulfilled.

OWEN H. WANGENSTEEN, *Journal of the*
American Medical Association, 1968

I returned to Red Surgery as the chief resident to start my final year of residency training in July 1965. I now had no scheduled night call, but I was on call every night for any problem on my service. No vacation time was allotted to a chief resident. I was expected to be available twenty-four hours a day 365 days of the year, the only exception being an out-of-town trip to present a paper at a scientific meeting.

How times have changed. Currently, chief residents take personal vacations, and, male or female, are granted additional time off for the arrival of a newborn. Clinical junior residents arrange their vacations among themselves and the department office at a time convenient for the resident, without any consultation with the chief resident or the head of the service the junior is assigned to.

They simply inform the service of their plans a week or even days before starting their vacation. In the past, junior residents could take vacation time only if granted by the service's chief resident and the attending head of the service. These arrangements were predicated on the needs of the service, not on the desires of the resident. I make no value judgment; I am simply recording facts.

During this rotation, Rich Lillehei and I worked extremely well together. He was a good mentor; he allowed me great freedom coupled with responsibility in running the service, and he provided me with substantial operating room experience as the operating surgeon. Our bond strengthened, and I am certain that this rotation was cardinal in Rich's accepting me as junior staff on Red Surgery about a year later.

During these four months, I became aware that Rich Lillehei was continuously challenging and provoking Richard Varco. I believe he did so because he resented Varco's eminence and arrogance and, even more so, his total command of the field of surgery and all related disciplines. Varco had come by his all-encompassing knowledge through continuous reading, listening to all presentations at surgical meetings, and, of course, his innate intelligence and capacity for original reasoning. Rich thought that he was equally well read, intelligent, and even more inventive. Therefore, at every Saturday conference, the weekly Tuesday complication conference, and surgery department or medical school lectures, Rich would rise to contradict or to provoke Richard Varco, who was easily provoked and loved a good fight. After his usually brilliant defensive argument, Varco would accelerate the rancor by an offensive, and at times personal, attack. Rich would retaliate and, if beaten in context and analysis, resort to cutting humor at Varco's expense. Rich usually drew a laugh from the audience and a frown from Varco. In wit, Rich had Varco beat, until the time Varco retorted that every court required a jester or court fool. Rich flushed with anger, and Varco, entirely apart from the merits of the argument at hand, won the joust for the day. No other staff members entered these contests on either side, and Wangensteen sat silently smiling, proud of them both. The rest of us were amused during these conferences and argued the opposing points of view afterward. These encounters enhanced our knowledge base, as well as our capacity for deductive reasoning and open intellectual combat.

My subsequent four-month rotation on Orange Surgery and, for that matter, the next eight months were eventful and life-changing. Richard Varco had requested me as his chief resident. Richard and I were transitioning into a lasting friendship, and he was instrumental in making my laboratory years a success. Varco took on the staff risk and protection for the first partial ileal bypasses, which I had performed as a laboratory resident two years short of completing the residency program. He endorsed me for fellowship in the prestigious surgical societies. At a later date, we received the $60 million Program on the Surgical Control of the Hyperlipidemias (POSCH) grant from the NIH because of his support and his contacts. He introduced me to, and facilitated my relationship with, the great surgeons of our time. He probably had my back on many occasions I was never even aware of. He was always my mentor. Whereas most residents and staff tried to avoid him, I sought him out. His intellectual guidance influenced my entire career. On all of our basic science lipid papers and all of the POSCH papers we published, I made him my coauthor. It was during this chief residency rotation that, securing his permission, I began to address him as Richard rather than Dr. Varco.

Just prior to my Orange Surgery chief residency rotation, Richard cut the median nerve in his right forearm. As I have mentioned, he was a cook and a baker. While baking bread one day, he shook a glass jar holding a yeast preparation. The jar exploded, and a sliver of glass cut his median nerve, which controls most of the motor and sensory functions of the hand. After several reparative attempts, immobilization by splint or cast, and two years of patient waiting, his nerve function recovered sufficiently for him to venture a return to the operating room. He was still a good technical surgeon but no longer the extraordinary surgeon that he had been. In his own mind, I believe that his performance fell below his acceptable standard for himself. I believe his injury was instrumental in hastening his fairly early retirement several years later.

Richard's nerve injury had a profound impact on me professionally. I was now chief resident on the rotation that I had looked forward to all my residency years, and this should have been my opportunity to operate with him for four months. But Richard could not operate. This did not prevent him from seeing patients, consulting, accepting referrals, and running a full operating-room schedule. His heart cases fell under the responsibility of Aldo Castaneda, at that time on the faculty before he moved to Children's Hospital in Boston. I was to do all other cases with a staff surgeon of my choosing if I wanted senior assistance. I was free to request aid from anyone, as long as it was not Rich Lillehei, whom Varco forbade me to call in.

One day I asked Ward Griffen, who was comparable in skill as a surgeon to Aldo Castaneda and was now on the attending faculty, to help me with a graft replacement of a large, expanding abdominal aortic aneurysm. The operation itself went well. Ward and I were satisfied with our efforts even though the patient's native artery was quite atherosclerotic and, therefore, not the best tissue to hold sutures. Given the situation, we did the best that we could. On postoperative night two, I received an emergency call from the junior resident on call. Our patient was bleeding, his abdomen was rapidly distending, and he was in shock. I knew he had ruptured a pseudoaneurysm (a ballooned-out area of an artery) at a suture site. I had seen a similar case on Rich Lillehei's service. Rich's patient had bled out on the ward. I told the junior resident to rush the patient to the operating room, pump in blood, and call Ward Griffen. I raced the twelve miles from home to the hospital, hoping to be stopped by a police car that would escort me to the hospital, but the only attention I attracted was that of a youngster who thought I wanted to race. Ward, who lived closer to the hospital in St. Paul, was already in the operating room when I arrived. We were, however, too late. Ward and I told Richard Varco of the patient's death the next morning. He looked at us and said, "The man is dead," and walked away. I felt deeply and personally responsible. Without the initial surgical intervention two days earlier, this man would have died by a spontaneous rupture of his severely diseased aorta. Yet, my role as the co-surgeon was to prevent his death, not to accelerate it. I will never forget this patient and that night.

During these four months on Orange Surgery, I asked Richard many times to come into the operating room with me, to scrub in, to criticize, and to guide me verbally. He always refused. One day, I had a Whipple procedure on the schedule and I said to Richard that I was confident doing the operation, but at least once during these four months, I would like him to be in the operating room with me. He consented but refused to scrub in and stood behind the anesthesia screen. A Whipple operation for cancer of the head of the pancreas involves a massive resection of pancreas, stomach, and segments of the small intestine in the hope of achieving a cure. Throughout the case, Varco would grunt from time to time. I asked him why he grunted. He said, never mind, go on and operate. Thus, I finished the case with no affirmative, negative, or helpful commentary from Richard, only grunts. I thought I had done the operation quite well. I walked out of the operating room with Richard and went fishing for a compliment. What a mistake! All I received was another grunt. I pressed the issue, asking him for a critique. He looked at me and said, "I'm letting you do my cases. That should be enough for you."

In 1953, Richard Varco did the first jejunoileal bypass operation for morbid obesity—taking more than 90 percent of the small intestine out of contact with food and, thereby, caloric absorption. He never published this case. The first four cases were published by John Linner and Arnold Kremen from our department in 1954. These surgeons subsequently left the university for private practice in Minneapolis. In 1966, the jejunoileal bypass operation was coming into greater use, and Richard, ever the visionary, wanted us to enter the field of bariatric surgery. He asked me, over and over again, to start doing jejunoileal bypasses. I steadfastly refused, saying that my name would become associated with obesity surgery rather than with my work in the lipid/atherosclerosis field. Further, the partial ileal bypass, not a weight-losing operation and already associated with my name, would be confused with the jejunoileal bypass.

One day, I was walking down the hallway of the Heart Hospital and ran into Richard, who had just had a new cast applied to his right forearm to facilitate median nerve regrowth by immobilization. He was in a dark mood. He accosted me and said that he had seen a perfect patient for a jejunoileal bypass. I again refused to do the operation. Varco waved his casted right arm at me, angrily exclaiming, "If I could operate, I would do it. I ask you to do it for us, and you refuse me." I immediately relented, and in 1966 did my first jejunoileal bypass. I was right: my name became associated with bariatric surgery. However, I have no regrets. Indeed, as I became more and more acquainted with the problem of morbid obesity and the unfortunate individuals suffering from this disease, the more grateful I was to Richard for forcing me to become involved, and very rapidly I became dedicated to the discipline. Thus, as I completed my residency, I was already intimately engaged in two of the cardinal areas of my career—lipids/atherosclerosis and morbid obesity and its comorbidities.

During this rotation on Orange Surgery, my friendship with Varco deepened. We often traveled together to meetings, and these airplane trips remained a continuous surgery board examination. We roomed together as well. We once shared a room at the Francis Drake Hotel in San Francisco for a meeting of the American College of Surgeons. Richard preferred this hotel to the more exclusive Fairmont or others on top of Nob Hill because it was located opposite an unpretentious cafeteria that served a fabulous cantaloupe for breakfast. The evening before I was to give a presentation at the Surgical Forum of the college, I ate a sandwich and retired to our room to practice my talk. I was still young and not inclined to go out for a dinner and wine or an evening in the banjo bars on Broadway the night before I gave a talk. Richard went to dinner with some of his friends. About 8 p.m., the phone rang. A young man asked to speak to Richard about applying for a cardiovascular fellowship at Minnesota. I told him that Dr. Varco was out and would not return until late. I advised him to seek out Varco the next day. I told him that Varco would be at my lecture, dressed in his usual blue suit, and that I would introduce him. At about 10 p.m., the young man called again. I told him that Varco had not returned and that he should not call again that evening but wait to see Varco the following day. Richard came in around 11 p.m. and I informed him of the calls I had answered for him.

We were both asleep by midnight when the phone rang. Because the surgery service was covered, no one from the hospital would call either of us at midnight. We assumed that there must be some urgent problem with one of our families. Richard reached the telephone on the bedstand before I did. It was the same persistent young man. Richard signaled to me that it was not an urgent family matter and spoke calmly with the caller. I expected him to explode in rage, but he did not. Instead, he advised the young man that he, too, was eager to meet, and that he should wait for him in the lobby of the hotel at 5:30 a.m., because he, Varco, always took a walk at that time. When Richard got off the phone, I said to him, "You never walk at 5:30 in the morning." He responded, "You know that. I know that. But he does not know that."

We got up around seven o'clock and took turns washing and shaving. We dressed and headed down to the lobby. We saw a person, presumably the eager young man, asleep on a couch. I volunteered to wake him. Richard stopped me, saying, "I don't believe he has the stamina for a cardiovascular fellowship. Let's go have our melon." We never saw or heard from the young man again.

Eating out with Richard was often a unique experience and generally fun. He loved to eat well, and, if he liked a dish, he would eat a lot of it. As visible evidence of his appetite, he was rotund. His taste in food was for hearty fare. He loved to take us to Kramarczuk's, a Polish delicatessen a short drive from the university, which featured Polish, Italian, and other sausages, stuffed peppers, pierogi, and similar delicacies. We stood in line in the restaurant section of Kramarczuk's, were served cafeteria style, and then retired to a table to eat, at times sharing a table with strangers. In later years, when Richard lived in Canada and returned to the Twin Cities only for Christmas, it was my job to find a new restaurant for ethnic food that was free of pretentiousness, or we would return to Kramarczuk's.

I remember eating with Richard in a somewhat more upscale restaurant in Los Angeles. The meal was mediocre, bordering on bad. He said, "Watch this. I'll complain to the maître d' and he will not hear me." He called over the maître d' and, in a calm voice, said, "This was one of the worst meals I have ever eaten." The maître d' bowed, smiled, and responded, "Oh, thank you, sir, thank you." Richard looked at me and said, "See, what did I tell you?" As we left,

he completed my gustatory education by stating that it was important to eat a bad meal every so often in order to recognize a good
one.

On December 23, 1965, our Claire Gretchen was born by a
planned cesarean section. Daisy and I were greatly relieved that
there were no adverse events associated with this pregnancy.
Claire's middle name was given in honor of Gretchen Bloch, one
of the kindest persons we have ever known. After spending the first
months in our bedroom, we transformed the "sewing room" cubicle into Claire's room. Jane and Amy occupied the other second-
floor bedroom, sleeping in a double-decker bunk bed with Jane
on the top bunk. When my parents visited, they slept on a pullout
couch in the living room. When Daisy's parents visited, they rented
a room in a nearby motel.

After Claire's birth, my parents came to visit. My father had
begun seeing Dr. Naip Tuna for his periodic cardiac assessments.
After a snowstorm, one of many that winter, and, in order to keep
his appointment with Dr. Tuna, my father crawled out of the utility
room window because the door was blocked by snow. At that time,
my mother became concerned about Jane and Amy being trapped
in their upstairs room in the event of a fire. We therefore purchased
and installed a rope ladder to the frame of their window. We had
practice drills with Jane and Amy, which they enjoyed, letting the
ladder fall to the ground and exiting via the window.

In March 1966, I moved on to my final chief residency rotation
on Purple Surgery. Again, I was fated not to have an operating head
of service. Dr. Wangensteen had developed a severe case of periarte-
ritis nodosa, a debilitating disease of arteries with severe pain and
exhaustion, which he blamed on inoculations he received before
going on an overseas trip. He was placed on massive doses of ste-
roids; and early on in his illness, he was confined to bed by severe
weakness. He, like Varco, continued to run an active surgical ser-

vice, and, as in the preceding four months, I did most of the surgery. I reported to Dr. Wangensteen by phone every evening, usually starting our conversation with an inquiry on how he was faring. I remember one particular response early in my rotation. He said, "I have made great progress, Henry. I needed to be in bed twenty-four hours per day; I am now confined to bed for only twenty-three." When he improved somewhat and started to come into the office, he had a cot placed in it so he could take an afternoon nap. He never operated again. Although he recovered, he was forced to retire by the age regulations of the time. Actually, he extended his tenure by a few years by lying about his age.

Shortly after starting my Purple Surgery rotation, Dr. Wangensteen gave me a special assignment. A staff doctor had somehow managed to finish the residency program and was running, in admirable fashion, a detection center. He had never wanted to be an operating surgeon, recognizing that he was emotionally unsuited for the operating room and that he lacked the necessary dexterity. Yet, Dr. Wangensteen wanted him to be board-certified credentialed before he settled into his leadership capacity in disease detection, never again to enter an operating room. He had passed the written board exam, but before he could take the oral examination he needed to be involved in a certain number of specific operative cases. Dr. Wangensteen assigned the requisite number of cases to him and assigned me to take him through them. I stated that I should not be responsible for teaching basic surgery to a member of the faculty. Dr. Wangensteen duly noted my objection and told me to get on with it.

I started each of these cases, did the difficult dissection and laid it out for him to finish before paging him to the operating room. Even then he would not come immediately, instead sending word that he was occupied but would arrive shortly. When he arrived, he would scrub for well over the required ten minutes. Enter-

ing the operating room, he would often contaminate himself and
then excuse himself to rescrub. Whenever he actually stepped up
to the operating table, he would look at the field and declare that
he believed I had the situation well in hand and would not require
any further help from him. With that, I would finish the case. Later,
when Dr. Wangensteen asked how the operation went, I would give
him the details. Dr. Wangensteen submitted his name to take the
oral board examination. He never practiced surgery.

I made certain that during all my chief residency services, we
were prepared for Saturday conference. We would meet before or
after morning rounds, and I would review the junior residents' presentations and ascertain the knowledge base of the service's residents, interns, and students. One Saturday morning early in April
1966, I and my Purple Surgery house staff entered the second-floor
amphitheater where for generations Saturday morning conference
was held. There was something strange about the assembled group:
only residents and students were present. There was no staff except
for Joe Aust. He stood in the pit of the amphitheater next to a table
spread with stapled sets of pages and blue test booklets. He asked
all the residents to be seated, and he dismissed all the students. He
stated, with a grin, that we were going to be given a surprise test.
Without much thought, I reacted by standing up and stating that
this surprise test was inappropriate. I argued that the faculty had
every right to hold an examination but not to spring it on us when
we had worked hard to prepare cases and presentations for the
expected Saturday conference. I went on to say that this was not a
mature manner in which to treat the adult men (there were as yet
no women surgical residents) who cared for, and were responsible for, the faculty's patients. I stated that these were men in their
thirties, with families, who were, for the most part, armed services
veterans. Joe, in essence, told me to be quiet and sit down. Instead,
I continued my insurrection by stating that I would not take the

test and that I was leaving. I invited those who felt as I did to follow me. I walked down the steps of the amphitheater, exchanged harsh looks with Joe, and exited via the amphitheater pit door. I stood in the hallway for several minutes, waiting to see who would follow me. No one did. I went home. If transported back in time into the body of my thirty-four-year old self, would I do the same thing? Possibly. Probably!

The following Monday, I was scrubbed, doing one of Dr. Wangensteen's cases, when Joe Aust walked into the operating room and said that Dr. Wangensteen wanted to see me. I replied that I would see him as soon as I could reasonably leave the case. He stated that he had assigned a staff surgeon to replace me, and that I was to go to Dr. Wangensteen's office immediately. I complied. His secretary, Mrs. Hans, showed me into the office of "The Chief." Dr. Wangensteen looked at me sternly and asked me to substantiate or deny the events of last Saturday as they had been related to him by Joe Aust. My actions, and even my words, had been accurately described. I confirmed Aust's account. As he continued to look sternly at me, Dr. Wangensteen said, "I cannot have a resident in open conflict with my attending staff. I cannot have a resident publicly defy the orders of the professor in charge of the residency program. You are, therefore, no longer a resident in this surgical program." I did not know what to say in response. I would have been relieved if, as in Mozart's opera *Don Giovanni,* the floor had opened up and the flames of hell had swallowed me. I was speechless and was about to get up and leave when Dr. Wangensteen continued: "I have, therefore, made you an instructor in the department, as of last Friday. Mrs. Hans has the appropriate paperwork for you to sign as you leave. Under those circumstances, I have no objection to a member of the faculty challenging another faculty member. Further, Mrs. Hans has additional paperwork for you to sign, if you so wish, making you an assistant professor on the first of July. I believe that you now have a case to get back to." His expression had become benevolent; there was the characteristic twinkle in his eye, and he smiled. I got up and said all I could think of at the moment: "Thank you." He waved me out. As I reached the door, he said, "Henry, will you now as an instructor and, because the department is short a chief resident, continue, as a favor to me, to fulfill the role of the Purple Surgery chief resident until the end of June?" All I could say was, "Yes, sir. Of course, sir. Thank you, sir." I signed the papers Mrs. Hans held out for me and hurried back to the sanctuary of the operating room to reflect on what had just happened.

Joe Aust came into my operating room a few minutes later. He was surprised to see me scrubbed and operating happily. He asked what had happened in Dr. Wangensteen's office. I believe he thought the outcome would be catastrophic for me and that I would plead with him to intercede. I said only that the meeting had been very interesting, and that it would be best if he asked Dr. Wangensteen about it. Joe and I never discussed the issue of the exam again.

✤ 14 ✤

Assistant Professor

*Not to know what happened
before we were born is always
to remain a child.*

MARCUS TULLIUS CICERO,
in Hannis Taylor, *Cicero: A Sketch
of His Life and Works*, 1918

I ended my residency and concurrent instructorship in July 1966 and became an assistant professor. As a graduation gift, Richard Varco gave me a pair of white shoes made of kangaroo leather with thick, corrugated, hard rubber soles and heels for the operating room. They looked special and gleamingly new in their whiteness, complemented by thick white laces. One day, Dr. Konald Prem, chair of Obstetrics and Gynecology, asked me to scrub in his room and remove a gallbladder. As I did so, I noticed movement under the operating-room table and then heard giggling. Konnie, both tall and large, had dipped a laparotomy pad in evacuated blood and was rapidly painting my new white shoes and laces red. He emerged from under the table. He said, laughing, that my shoes had now been properly baptized. After the case, I scrubbed the blood off as well as I could, thereby dulling the leather. I wore these shoes for about fifty years and never wore others in the operating room. The chief operating room nurse made me replace the

146

knotted laces about fifteen years ago. The shoes themselves, except for the rubber cushions, have fallen apart and are held together by their laces. If one looks carefully, remnants of the original blood ritual in the cracks of the remaining kangaroo hide are still visible. I plan to have these shoes bronzed.

I joined Aldo Castaneda on the faculty at the time that Ward Griffen was in the process of moving to Lexington, Kentucky. Drs. Wangensteen and Varco never fully accepted the fact that Aldo and I were no longer their residents. Although there were several junior staff in addition to the two of us, Wangensteen and Varco insisted that Aldo and I do most of the cases they brought into the house that they, because of their physical problems, were unable to perform. Aldo was responsible for the heart cases, and I would help him if I finished earlier; I did the gastrointestinal operations, and Aldo would help me when he had completed his cardiac workload. So it went for several months, until one day when Dr. Wangensteen called me into his office.

During my chief residency year, I sat for my preliminary surgical PhD exam concurrently with the final oral examination for my MS in biochemistry. The Department of Physiology was also represented because that discipline was my MS minor. The three-hour examination passed rapidly and, I must say, I found it fun. Fortunately, I was able to derive the Michaelis–Menten equation and was not asked to expand a soap bubble mathematically. After the exam, Dr. Wangensteen, who chaired the proceedings, told me he was disappointed in my lack of knowledge about historical surgical and basic science personalities. I promised to rectify this failing.

Thus, when I entered Dr. Wangensteen's office that day and he told me I was in arrears with respect to my PhD, I was somewhat confused. He stated that I had as yet not handed in my PhD thesis, which was to be about the laboratory work in support of partial ileal bypass. I told him I was working on the thesis and that the time allowed for its completion was essentially undefined. He agreed, but he stated that it should be completed now because he wanted to confer my degree upon me before his pending forced retirement. I told him I would accelerate my writing progress. He stated that he would help me by banning me from performing surgery until I submitted the requisite bound copies of my thesis. I strongly objected to being shut out of the operating room and argued that this would decrease his caseload unless he assigned his cases to someone else. He said that his cases would either have to wait or go elsewhere for surgery. He added that my completion of the PhD was more important than the surgery cases that would be lost from the schedule. He assured me that his decision was final and told me to go home and write.

All the laboratory and clinical work for my PhD was complete, but I had barely begun the formal writing up of the work in the standard PhD format. I had to compose and write out the rough copy myself; type up the clean copy, including the requisite equations; make my own tables and graphs; and compile my references and bibliography. I could type, but not that well. There were no self-correcting typewriters and not as yet such an item as a desktop computer. I had to correct mistakes with white-out correction fluid, or, if a page became too sloppy, I had to retype it. It took me eight weeks to complete the thesis. When I presented Dr. Wangensteen with a carbon paper copy of the thesis, he allowed me to return to surgery, even though the bound copies of the thesis would still be several weeks in preparation.

These eight weeks of writing were notable for two reasons. Weekly, Aldo would call me. First he would inquire, almost solicitously, about my progress. I would tell him I was working hard and ask how he was doing. At that point in our conversation, he would often explode into expletives, saying his workload now kept him in the operating room every day, many nights, and most weekends. I assured him I would rather be operating than writing, but this was of no comfort to him. He would end our conversation by telling me to write less and come back sooner.

I did not write less. I very much enjoyed chronicling my laboratory years and the pleasure of the writing process itself. Yet I did miss surgery. I was rescued by Dr. Stanley Goldberg, who had finished his residency before me and entered the emerging field of colorectal surgery as the partner of Dr. Howard Frykman, a superb technical surgeon, in private practice at Abbott Northwestern Hospital. Stan has always been generous and helpful, providing me with excellent counsel over the years. He and Dr. Frykman offered me the opportunity to scrub on and perform one or two colon cases on Friday mornings at Abbott. From them I learned fine 5/0 nylon suture technique for bowel anastomoses. (Most surgeons at the time were sewing bowel with thicker sutures.) On receiving this kind offer, I offered in return to help out with night calls. They refused, saying that I must work primarily on my thesis, and, that if Dr. Wangensteen ever found out about my clandestine trips to their operating room, he would kill all of us. I increased my surgical skills by working with them, and I maintained my sanity, forgoing the withdrawal symptoms my addiction to the operating room would have caused.

The thesis defense examination was actually a pleasant experience, because I realized that I should know more about my own research than anyone else in the room. (In later years, when I served as a PhD examiner, chaired PhD committees, and mentored and advised PhD candidates, I would always tell the candidates to relax, because if they were not the most knowledgeable person on their chosen subject in the room that day, they did not deserve a PhD.) I thought I had done somewhat better answering Dr. Wangensteen's surgical history questions, but when we walked out of the exam together, he again corrected my historical knowledge and told me what further information I should acquire and where to find it. I brought cookies and lemonade for the examiners, and, I believe, started a tradition of camaraderie and bribery.

Dr. Wangensteen submitted my PhD thesis, accompanied by reprints of my pertinent publications, for consideration for the Samuel D. Gross Prize. This prestigious national award is given by the Philadelphia Academy of Surgery in honor of its namesake, an internationally renowned cardiovascular and pediatric surgeon. I won the award, only the third recipient from Minnesota to receive this distinction. The first was Owen H. Wangensteen; the second was George E. Moore. At present, I am the last University of Minnesota Gross Prize awardee. I purchased a secondhand tuxedo. Daisy groomed me, and I went to Philadelphia for the formal dinner presentation.

Wangensteen was intent on finding positions outside Minnesota for his promising students. He wanted to seed American academic surgery with his trained disciples, surgeons who believed in the concept of the triple-threat academic surgeon, equal parts clinician, basic researcher, and educator. He tried to get both the Lilleheis to accept chairmanships elsewhere, but they successfully evaded him. He arranged for Varco to become the chair of surgery at the College of Physicians and Surgeons of Columbia University, but Richard refused to go.

He soon started on me, wanting me to take a bridge position as the chief of surgery of the department's academic unit at Mt. Sinai Hospital. He approached me one day, saying, "Henry, I want you to consider the position at Mt. Sinai." I said I would rather not. He insisted that I visit there, which I did. I was conducted around the hospital by Dr. Arnold Kremen, the best surgeon at the institution, who wanted to run the teaching unit and its residents, but without any ties to Dr. Wangensteen and the jurisdiction of our department. He was most uncordial and made it quite evident that I was not welcome. I reported back to Dr. Wangensteen and explained why I would not go to Mt. Sinai. "The Chief" left me alone for several weeks but then said to me that I was good enough and strong enough to survive in the unfriendly atmosphere of Mt. Sinai. He now addressed me only as Dr. Buchwald, instead of the familiar "Henry" he had used for years. I again refused to consider Mt. Sinai. He let several weeks pass and tried again, this time ordering me to represent our interest on the Mt. Sinai board of directors, which, of course, I had to do. On rounds and elsewhere, he now called me "Buchwald." I fought with Kremen on the board, though others at Mt. Sinai really wanted me to come and take the chief position. However, I saw no future for myself there. I again said no to Dr. Wangensteen, who was now addressing me only as "Doctor." Then, suddenly, Dr. Wangensteen's campaign was over. One day he smiled at me and said, "Henry, come to my office. I want to chat with you." I maintained my seat on the Mt. Sinai board, representing the university, and I was instrumental in having Dr. Cassius Ellis installed as the chief of surgery at Mt. Sinai. He made a splendid head of surgery, but eventually, also unhappy in the fractious atmosphere, he moved to North Memorial. At the time, though, I delighted in securing this position for Dr. Ellis, an outspoken African American surgeon who I had helped train.

In addition to our clinical workload, Dr. Wangensteen made Aldo the head of the residency program and me the head of the intern year and intern selection. I believe this "promotion" was punishment for my rebellion against Joe Aust, who was now chairman of surgery in San Antonio. Aldo and I organized the programs, imposing more definitive structure. When Aldo left, I inherited responsibility for the combined intern and residency program.

Thus, seven years after arriving in Minnesota as a surgical resident, I was an assistant professor in charge of the residency program. I was a laboratory and clinical researcher with independent funding. I believed myself to be a teacher and, as an academic, a lifelong student. I was American Board of Surgery certified. I realize that attaining these goals would not have been possible without the mentors who gave me their time, their erudition, their kindness, and their goodwill. These mentors included my attending staff, in particular Drs. Richard Varco, Owen Wangensteen, Richard Lillehei, Al Sullivan, and Joe Aust; my peers, especially Drs. Jack Bloch, Ward Griffen, Aldo Castaneda, Jack Delaney, and Don McQuarrie; and my laboratory coworkers, notably Marshall Schwartz, Josie Bertisch, Laurie Fitch, and Roger Gephart.

❧ 15 ❧

Endgame

*In summary, plant a tree for posterity
in the orchard of your profession.
It will give you enduring satisfaction
though you may never live to see
it mature; its growth can project your
image and wishes far into time
and space.*

OWEN H. WANGENSTEEN, *Journal of
the American Medical Association*,
1968

Thirty-seven years after he was appointed chair of the Department of Surgery of the University of Minnesota, Dr. Wangensteen retired, signifying the end of an era. Dr. John S. Najarian succeeded Dr. Wangensteen as department chair and ushered in a second epoch of national greatness in academic surgery, with particular emphasis in transplant surgery. Dr. Najarian relinquished the chair in 1993. For these sixty-one years, the reputation of the Department of Surgery as an engine for research, innovative surgery, and scholarship was unrivaled.

During my tenure in the Wangensteen era, 1960 to 1967, the Department of Surgery was at the zenith of its accomplishments and renown. The dazzling contributions of the department impacted the lives of millions of people throughout the world and changed the course of medicine in the twentieth century. As a coda to the Wangensteen era after 1967, I will outline the subsequent histories of seven of its principal surgeons who I knew well and worked with.

Dr. Joseph (Joe) Bradley (Brad) Aust left the Minnesota Department of Surgery in 1965 to become the chair of the new department of surgery at the fledgling University of Texas Medical School in San Antonio, Texas. Joe took with him two outstanding Minnesota surgeons—Dr. Harlan Root and Dr. Arthur McFee. All three had previously served in the U.S. Navy and preserved navy habits of no-nonsense discipline in their personal demeanor. Over thirty years, they built a department based on Wangensteen principles and made it the premier surgery institution in Texas and one of the best in the nation. Joe became president of three notable regional surgical societies: the Texas, the Western, and the Southern. He was also a prominent figure in the American Surgical Association. I will always remember Brad for his idiosyncratic handshake. Whenever I or others met him at a national meeting, he uttered a bellicose greeting and clasped your hand, exerting all his strength in a powerful grip until you capitulated by pleading the need to use your hand for performing surgery. He would then laugh and reminisce about old times. He died at the age of eighty-four.

My close friend Dr. Jack Bloch left the University of Minnesota with Dr. Walt Lillehei in 1968 for the Cornell Medical School, New York Hospital, to complete his cardiovascular surgery training. After Cornell and three years in the College of Medicine in Peoria, Illinois, he was recruited to become the chief of surgery at Kern Medical Center in Bakersfield, California, an affiliate of UCLA. He, too, made a lesser-known hospital into a first-class surgical program. A brilliant general and cardiovascular surgeon, he was the epitome of a teacher, in and out of the operating room. During his tenure as chair through 2005, and in his postretirement teaching position until 2014, he trained more than one hundred individuals to operate, to take excellent care of their patients, and, above all, to think in the Wangensteen tradition that all surgery is based on scholarship and research for the future. He was the most patient, kind, and understanding mentor who emerged from our common Minnesota roots. Jack died at the age of eighty-five in 2015. His wonderful wife, Gretchen, lives on. His two sons continue his love for the practice of medicine: Robert is a radiologist and Paul is a vascular surgeon.

Dr. Jack Delaney, though officially retired and on emeritus status, retained his laboratory into his mid-eighties, funded by a gift from a grateful patient. He explored and published research on preventing adhesions, that bête noir of surgery, and the use of prosthetic materials for hernia repairs. The Department of Surgery granted him a desk in the tiniest office to share with two other alumni professors, and he faithfully attended and participated in surgery grand rounds. He was selected for the honor of Alumnus of the Year; he spoke eloquently and honestly about the negative changes in academic freedom and the importance of research in a surgical education. Most of Jack's time in retirement was spent with his family—wife Puddy, children, and grandchildren. Daisy and I enjoyed seeing Jack and Puddy from time to time, sharing dinner and reminiscences, as well as talking of changing mores in current times. Jack died short of his ninetieth birthday, leaving us with this pithy saying: "I don't want to be ninety; nothing good happens after that."

Dr. Clarence (C.) Walton (Walt) Lillehei left Minnesota in 1967. It was inevitable that he would clash with Dr. John Najarian when he succeeded Wangensteen as chair. They were both alpha personalities who tolerated no incursion into their surgical domains. Further, it was well known that Wangensteen had advocated and campaigned for Walt Lillehei to replace him as chair. The selection committee, however, chose to go with the outsider, not the local and locally favored candidate. After that decision, Walt accepted the Lewis Atterbury Stimson professorship and chair of the Department of Surgery at Cornell Medical Center in New York City, taking most of his residents and fellows with him.

Walt had a large basic research laboratory at Minnesota, well funded by the National Institutes of Health (NIH). The lab contained expensive cardiovascular research equipment purchased with NIH grant money. Dr. Najarian told Walt that even though his NIH grant was transferable to Cornell, he could not take the equipment with him. The story is told that over a weekend, Walt hired a moving company to pack up all of his equipment. Walt left with the movers for New York. On Monday morning, when Dr. Najarian found out about this escapade, he called the Minnesota State Highway Patrol to intercept Lillehei; however, Lillehei and his caravan of moving vans had already crossed the Minnesota border into Wisconsin. Lillehei left a farewell gift for Najarian in the capacious and now totally empty laboratory space he had evacuated—a bedpan containing a rose.

During his tenure at Cornell, Walt Lillehei changed that institution's reputation from a destination for excellent surgery to that of a world center for the burgeoning field of cardiovascular surgery, as well as for surgical innovation and imaginative concepts.

Ever since his days of bioengineering with Earl Bakken and the invention of the cardiac pacemaker, Walt Lillehei remained interested in developing instrumentation for the medical device industry. In 1975, he returned to St. Paul, accepting the position of director of medical affairs for the St. Jude Company, concurrently with a clinical professorship at the University of Minnesota.

During these latter years, I saw Walt from time to time. We talked about inventions and how to facilitate their commercialization. I last saw him nine months before his death in 1999 at the age of eighty, at a gala birthday party given in his honor by his wife and family. He was as I always knew him—outgoing, keenly intelligent, fun-loving, advocating that life should be conducted with goodwill and humor.

Richard (Rich) Carlton (C.) Lillehei remained at the University of Minnesota for his entire surgical career. As Dr. Najarian loaded the surgery faculty with people of his choosing, mostly transplant surgeons, a cadre of Wangensteen faculty—Rich Lillehei, Richard Varco, Theodor Grage, Jack Delaney, Bob Goodale, and me—essentially represented the gastrointestinal, cardiovascular, pulmonary, breast, endocrine, cancer, head and neck, hernia, peripheral vascular, and bariatric disciplines. Rich, however, was also a transplant surgeon and had achieved fame for performing the world's first pancreas transplant and one of the first successful transplants of human intestine in a patient with shortgut syndrome. His relationship with Najarian was, therefore, also bound to be competitive, but, unlike the hostility between Najarian and Rich's older brother, Walt, he and John Najarian usually avoided open confrontation and managed to coexist.

Rich Lillehei was considered, in and out of Minnesota, to be a surgeon with great promise, a prodigy of surgery. By his fifties he was well known as a cardiovascular and transplant surgeon, an imaginative therapist in the treatment of shock, and a pioneer in organ preservation for transplantation. Unfortunately, his life was cut short at the age of fifty-three.

Walt Lillehei often stated that the heart had just so many beats and that he was not going to waste them on exercise. Not so for his brother Rich, who was an avid athlete. He skied, he skated, he played tennis, and he ran. As I mentioned earlier, once after a major snowstorm with all roads closed to traffic, Rich skied the five miles to the university for his morning case in surgery. Rich had run several marathons and was training for the Boston Marathon at his second home in Sanibel, Florida, when he died. After sailing all morning with his sons and, without resting and perhaps properly hydrating, he set out for a long practice run. His body was found on a beach, with death apparently from a cardiac dysrhythmia, possibly caused by a fluid/electrolyte imbalance.

Dr. Richard L. Varco, the mentor of mentors, lived a rich, contemplative life into his nineties. About two years after his median nerve injury and a prolonged interval of healing, Richard returned to the operating room, but he was not satisfied with his performance because he did not meet his own standard of perfection. He retired from the University of Minnesota in 1981 as a Regents' Professor, the highest honor bestowed on a member of the university faculty.

For his retirement, Varco had purchased an isolated ranch in Montana, his native state. He sold it in favor of a majestic hillside property on Halfmoon Bay, a peninsula in Canada, reachable by ferry from Vancouver. It was there that he designed his and Louise's retirement home and garden, landscaped the hillside leading to the bay, and lived for the final twenty-five years of his unique life. I asked him why he had changed his choice of retirement haven from Montana to Canada. He said he did not mind dying suddenly from a stroke or heart attack but was concerned that Louise might be faced with disposing of his body in a remote snowy wasteland, or, if he survived the initial event, he was concerned that she might be burdened by an incapacitated man in desolate country. He chose, therefore, a more inhabited, yet still wild, area with a nearby hospital.

Daisy and I visited Richard and Louise in Halfmoon Bay and stayed at their home. The living room, a comfortable room for reading, faced the wilderness with a view of the bay, with a large stone fireplace on the other side. His was a chef's kitchen with a walk-in freezer where he stored venison and other meats. During our visit, he spent mornings working his many acres of bamboo and indigenous trees, sculpting vistas for viewing the land and the sea. I caught an image of him on camera emerging from working his primeval woodland, a beatific smile on his face. His garden was vast and contained vegetables and row upon row of red flowers, mostly rhododendrons. One morning, I rose early and went outside to find Richard, who had risen even earlier, on his knees tending to his plants. I sipped on a cup of coffee and did not speak. Richard looked up and said, "I suppose you are going to ask me why I have so many red flowers?" I did not respond; I knew he would answer his own question sooner or later, whether I asked or not. He said, "Because I like red flowers."

Varco parted with the University of Minnesota administration on acrimonious terms, a scenario more common than not at academic institutions. Aged surgeons beyond their years of providing revenue to the university coffers cease to be institution favorites. Richard donated several million dollars to the university, as had some of his family members. In making this gift, he specified that it should be used for teaching and for aiding residents in their research endeavors. Instead, the university, stating that all university uses were for education, used his gift for everything but Richard's intended wishes. After years of quarreling, appealing to the university president, and taking legal action, Richard lost his battle to specify the use of his donated money. From observing similar disputes, I realized that a university donor could prevail in a dispute over the distribution of moneys only if he or she promised additional future gifts.

In 1996, Richard came to Minneapolis pale and barely able to walk, with a staggeringly low hemoglobin value between 3.0 and 4.0 g/dL (normal 12–14 g/dL). He asked me to take care of him. I admitted him to the hospital, transfused him to a normal hemoglobin, and determined that he was suffering from an unusual case of jejunal diverticulitis populated by iron-eating bacteria. A prolonged course of antibiotic therapy was curative. I mention this episode in Richard's life because it illustrated his enduring personality. There was not a day during his hospitalization that he did not tell me what to do, usually favoring a surgical solution, but ending his long display of erudition and suggestions with the statement that, "Of course, you are in charge."

In May 2004, at the age of ninety-one, Richard died of pneumonia at the rural hospital in Halfmoon Bay. His wife Louise continued to live an active life in Halfmoon Bay and Minneapolis until the age of ninety-eight. I stay in touch with some of Richard's seven children from whom I received a one-of-a-kind collection of films of the earliest open-heart operations. I had these milestones in the history of medicine digitized and donated them to the University of Minnesota archives in the Elmer Andersen Library for future generations to relive, wonder at, and be inspired by. Outside the province of the University of Minnesota, the Varco family established the Richard and Louise Varco student scholarship to encourage young people to pursue higher education. This gift will allow other youngsters to aspire to become a Richard Varco.

Owen Wangensteen, the intellectual parent of the Minnesota surgery dynasty, did not wish to retire from the work he loved. In the 1960s, the federal mandate forbidding ageism in government-supported institutions was as yet not in effect, and the University of Minnesota had a mandatory retirement policy effective at the age of sixty-five. Wangensteen managed to hold on until the age of sixty-seven, when he was forced not only to relinquish the chair of surgery but to accept emeritus status.

Owen's wife, Sarah (called Sally), confided to me that Owen's successor, John Najarian, told Owen that he was no longer welcome at the Saturday morning grand rounds he had initiated. Najarian wanted grand rounds to be his exclusive domain. He stated to Owen that he should satisfy his desire for academic discourse by attending rounds at the VA Hospital surgery affiliate. Wangensteen knew that Najarian needed to start his own tradition and decided that he was not going to be an obstacle in his path. As long as Najarian maintained excellence and departmental emphasis on training academic surgeons, Wangensteen offered him his support with no outward demonstration of displeasure or grievance. Najarian had Wangensteen's fifth-floor Mayo Building office suite destroyed and inaugurated a departmental floor containing his own elaborate office on the eleventh floor of the newly named Phillips-Wangensteen Building. During his entire tenure as chairman, John Najarian resided in the Wangensteen Building.

Wangensteen was well recognized in his lifetime for his many achievements, including authorship of about nine hundred peer-reviewed publications. The dozens of honors he received include the Samuel D. Gross Award from the Philadelphia Academy of Science; election to the U.S. National Academy of Sciences; Honorary Fellowship in the Royal College of Surgeons of England, as well as that of Edinburgh and Ireland, and several other nations; presidency of the American Surgical Association; and presidency of the American College of Surgeons. He was named in many a dedication in texts of surgery. He was revered as the greatest teacher of surgery of the twentieth century.

Wangensteen never lost his academic interests, especially in the education of surgical residents. He attended all the sessions he could of the American College of Surgeons' Surgical Forum, now renamed the Owen H. Wangensteen Surgical Forum. I sat with him during one such session as a paper coauthored by his son Steve was being introduced. There were two residents from another institution seated in front of us. On reading the program, one said to his companion, "Wangensteen? I thought he was dead." I told Dr. Wangensteen that I would go over and introduce him to them. Wangensteen said, "Don't do that, Henry. The shock might be too much for them."

In retirement, Wangensteen was free to pursue his avocations of giving the craft of surgery a history and a place in the medical school and surgical residency curriculum, writing for posterity, and bird-watching. He shared these enterprises with his wife, also a medical historian and the former editor of *Minnesota Medicine*. Wangensteen became a bird-watcher because Sally loved it. Sally was the greatest gift bestowed on Owen. Together, Owen and Sally organized and raised the funds for the Wangensteen Historical Library of Biology and Medicine on the fifth floor of Diehl Hall, as well as the stipend for a permanent position for a medical historian. When at the university, they worked in a small office next to this library. They coauthored a magisterial 785-page tome, published by the University of Minnesota Press in 1979: *The Rise of Surgery: From Empiric Craft to Scientific Discipline*. The carefully chosen title clearly expresses the perceptive philosophy of its authors. This gigantic volume gives dates, names, places, and insights into fascinating personalities. It is a go-to book for any surgeon interested in the roots of his or her calling.

On January 13, 1981, Owen Wangensteen was at home editing a paper when he sustained a fatal heart attack. He was eighty-two years old.

Many offshoots sprang from the Wangensteen root system—surgeons who altered the lives of hundreds of thousands of patients, contributed to scientific knowledge and medical care, led programs in the training of various surgical crafts, and served as exemplars in their professional and personal communities. Of the approximately five hundred graduates of the Wangensteen PhD program, many were responsible for significant contributions in communities throughout the United States and elsewhere.

On any given day, a farmer in Tuscany, Italy, will be treated for a bowel obstruction by Wangensteen suction, a young child in China will have an imperfect heart repaired with ease, the lessons of organ transplantation will allow special teams of surgeons in the United States to transplant a human face, and the world epidemic of obesity will be challenged by bariatric surgery. These procedures and many others, and the knowledge to undertake them, originated and were facilitated and disseminated by the Minnesota heritage in surgery.

An important part of this heritage is the perpetuation of the Wangensteen residency program tradition. Many departments of surgery have instituted basic research years as part of their residency programs, programs that teach young surgeons to think not only clinically, but innovatively, in a tradition of free expression and interdisciplinary exchange of knowledge and cooperative endeavors.

Unfortunately, preservation of past excellence is selective and difficult in medicine and science, particularly so in continuing to recognize the giants who created that history. While the public can name Einstein; few, if any, can name Billroth, Carel, Wangensteen, and other standouts of his era. The world takes their accomplishments for granted—the patients saved from death, the hearts mended, the longevity bestowed—without any knowledge of the lives, travails, and triumphs of these pioneers of medicine.

In preceding chapters I have cited surgical milestones of the Wangensteen era. They include ascertaining the etiology and therapy for intestinal obstruction; earliest open-heart surgery; heart transplantations; invention of the bubble pump oxygenator; invention of the implantable cardiac pacemaker; the first bariatric surgery procedure; the first pancreas transplant; pioneering efforts in bowel transplantation and organ preservation; and landmark concepts in the treatment of shock. These were cardinal contributions to health care. There were in addition many other major innovations stemming from the Wangensteen era and its perpetuation by his disciples.

Most of the Wangensteen-era surgeons were in the various armed services for a minimum of two years, in times of both war and relative peace. These years undoubtedly gave us not only a sense of allegiance to our country but a perspective for what is important and what is not. They strengthened our sense of independence and our resilience in the face of adversity. And, during these years, each of us contributed practical concepts to the military, some of which have survived the test of time.

Metabolic/Bariatric Surgery

In my own area of work, metabolic/bariatric surgery, I mentioned the first bariatric operation in 1953 by Dr. Richard L. Varco. A great deal of the subsequent history of this discipline is intimately linked to Minnesota and the Wangensteen heritage. Dr. Edward E. Mason, long considered the father of bariatric surgery, trained at the University of Minnesota. He then joined the faculty of the University of Iowa, where he accomplished his pioneering work in the field. In 1966, Mason and Dr. Chikashi Ito published their trailblazing paper on gastric bypass. In 1977, Dr. John F. Alden, also a product of the Department of Surgery of the University of Minnesota, introduced cross-stapling of the stomach to gastric bypass, thereby eliminating the need for gastric division. In the same year, Dr. Ward O. Griffen, a graduate of the Minnesota program, having now assumed the position of Chair of Surgery at the University of Kentucky, reported the first gastric bypass with a Roux-en-Y gastrojejunostomy (joining of the upper gastric pouch of a gastric bypass to an isolated limb of jejunum). This was the progenitor of the classic gastric bypass procedure.

Gastroplasty, the isolation of a restricted segment of the stomach to produce early satiety and thereby weight loss, was first introduced by Dr. Kenneth J. Printen and Mason in 1973. Mason's modification, in 1982, of the vertical banded gastroplasty became the dominant operation in the field in the late 1980s through the early 1990s.

Fecal Transplantation

Fecal transplantation can be defined as the transfer of normal stool by mouth, upper gastrointestinal tube, enema, and currently in capsules, to introduce healthy gut microbiota into a bowel infected with unhealthy microorganisms responsible for *clostridium difficile* syndrome and other pathogenic gastrointestinal conditions. Historically, Chinese writings seven hundred years ago credit the use of fecal transplantation by mouth to Ge Hong, a practitioner of holistic medicine. The first modern literature on fecal transplantation by enema was authored in 1958 by Dr. Benjamin (Ben) Eiseman and associates, published in Dr. Wangensteen's journal *Surgery*.

In 1961, during my first Purple Surgery rotation, a man was admitted to our service with intractable diarrhea, abdominal pain, and weight loss. He was failing rapidly. Our administration of intravenous fluids, antispasmodics, and many other agents proved ineffective in halting his progress to fatality. One day on patient rounds, Dr. Wangensteen suggested that this man must have bad bacteria in his gut that might be suppressed by the introduction of good intestinal organisms. He turned to us, his resident retinue, and instructed us to insert a nasogastric (Wangensteen) tube, and administer a large quantity of normal feces via the tube. I naively asked, "Where are we to obtain the feces, Dr. Wangensteen?" He winked at me and said, "Use your imagination, Henry, use your imagination." We generated the required material, made it into a slurry, and followed Dr. Wangensteen's instructions. The man fully recovered and left the hospital. We were the first, therefore, to utilize fecal transplantation in Minnesota and probably the first to employ upper gastrointestinal gavage to do so.

Pediatric Cancer

Dr. Arnold Leonard has had a far-reaching impact on pediatric surgery and the treatment of pediatric cancers. His original research into the modification of salmonella bacteria rendering it nontoxic but capable of penetrating and killing cancer cells continues to be a highly promising line of genetic engineering investigation. His contributions have impacted the treatment of Wilms tumor and cystic fibrosis in children; he developed the modern method for treating congenital collapsed chest deformity (pectus excavatum); and he invented several gastrointestinal and intravenous access catheters in common use today.

Functional Liver Contributions

In 1960, Dr. Henry Gans, while in the Minnesota Department of Surgery, introduced the first anticlotting agents as lifesaving treatment for excessive bleeding associated with liver and open-heart operation. Dr. Gans's most monumental contribution was the detailing of the anatomy of the human liver, accurately depicting its structures, vessels, and bile ducts, which served as the foundation for subsequent liver resections and transplantations. Based on this knowledge, he performed the world's first two split-liver transplants, when he moved to New York's Cornell University Medical Center, in 1969.

Extension of Pediatric Cardiovascular Surgery

By the 1960s, pediatric cardiovascular surgery was flourishing. In 1958, at the Mayo Clinic, surgeons were investigating the use of arteriovenous fistulas (conduits) between the femoral artery and the femoral vein in the upper thigh to achieve increased blood flow to the lower extremity, in order to equalize leg length in children left with stunted leg growth after polio. Richard Varco, with myself in tow, modified this procedure, and we performed several such operations at the local Shriners Hospital for Children in St. Paul, albeit with equivocal results.

When in 1972, Dr. Aldo Castaneda left Minnesota to start his own legacy in pediatric cardiovascular surgery at Boston's Children's Hospital, he was imbued with the Minnesota philosophy of innovation, striving to do what had been deemed impossible. He was also blessed with the technical brilliance to initiate these tasks. He soon became known as the father of neonatal pediatric cardiac surgery. He was the first to switch the aorta and pulmonary arteries emanating from the heart to treat congenital transposition of the great vessels, and the first to perform a one-stage complete repair of the tetralogy of Fallot, a highly complicated congenital malformation of the heart, previously only approached by staged procedures. In addition, in the Wangensteen tradition, he trained hundreds of pediatric cardiovascular surgeons.

Cardiac Catheterization

Cardiac catheterization was initiated by Drs. Andre Cournand and Dickinson Richards at Bellevue Hospital in New York in the 1940s, using each other to test their concept and instruments. Selective coronary arteriography was first described by Dr. F. Mason Sones of the Cleveland Clinic in the 1960s. Yet these procedures were not practiced or advocated by cardiologists, pediatricians, and radiologists at the University of Minnesota. Dr. Walt Lillehei tried inviting these medical colleagues to join his cardiac surgery program and perform these services—to no avail. Walt, in typical Minnesota Department of Surgery fashion, said, "We will do it ourselves." Thus, he and many of the resident staff performed the original cardiac catheterizations at Minnesota. This procedure was done in addition to surgery and bedside clinical care, often utilizing most of the twenty-four hours in a given day. After the successful establishment of a cardiac catheterization program by surgery, Dr. Kurt Amplatz, a Minnesota pioneer of invasive radiology, assumed responsibility for these procedures. During his long tenure at Minnesota, Dr. Amplatz became well recognized as an inventor of invasive radiology instrumentation and the procedures for its utilization.

Dedicated Intensive-Care Unit and Parenteral Nutrition

The intensive-care unit (ICU) concept for patients with severe or life-threatening illnesses or injuries was promulgated in the 1950s. By the 1960s, there was an ICU (station 44) at the University Hospital, located on the fourth floor, down a hallway from the operating room. There were, however, no intensive-care specialists or fellows. Postoperative care was the sole responsibility of the surgical service performing the surgery. Thus, the residency staff at night covered not only the general floor patients but the ICU patients as well. Under Walt Lillehei, Rich Lillehei, and Richard Varco, the expertise and specialization of the ICU nursing staff was prioritized and proved essential to the success of open-heart and other complicated operative procedures. Also, in particular under the aegis of Rich Lillehei, resuscitation of the patient in cardiovascular collapse from shock was studied and its therapy markedly improved.

Total parenteral hyperalimentation, introduced by Dr. Stanley J. Dudrick at the University of Pennsylvania in the 1960s, was adopted at Minnesota and became a major therapeutic for patients unable to sustain oral nutrition. However, well before the advent of commercial nontoxic intravenous formulas of nutrients, vitamins, and minerals for total nutrition, we at Minnesota were testing various intravenous hyperalimentation solutions high in their concentrations of protein and fat to be used as supplements or partial replacement of oral nutrition. These studies contributed knowledge to the standardization of intravenous alimentation throughout the country. In later years, under the aegis of Dr. Frank Cerra, Minnesota pioneered the employment of home total parenteral nutrition, providing patients freedom from hospitalization.

Academic Surgery

The ultimate aim of the Wangensteen program was to make the academic surgeon an innovator, a basic as well as a clinical researcher, and a scholar. All surgeons were to be thinkers as well as doers. We were to spread this gospel and thereby reform and reshape American surgery. To a great extent, we have been successful. We started in the prototype idea factory, developed the satellite institutions, and maintained the heritage. The challenge for the foreseeable future will be to honor and practice the concept of the idea factory and the joy of participating in its work.

Epilogue

Have I lived hopefully?

THE TALMUD, Tractate Shabbat

This retrospective of an era is written from my reflections, memories, and assessment of people and events. For the reader to understand my mindset, I provided information about my life prior to coming to Minnesota in 1960; I conclude with an epilogue of my life after 1967.

Since the time of the peripatetic monk-scholars of the Middle Ages in Europe who traveled from city to city and university to university, academics, in particular medical-school clinical academics, have been wanderers in their quest for advancement and for opportunity. Opportunities were abundantly open to me at the University of Minnesota, and so, in spite of academic offers elsewhere, I remained there. I can honestly say that my career goals have been those embodied in the Wangensteen tradition: to be a clinical surgeon, a researcher, a teacher, and a scholar.

In the spring and summer seasons, during the time we lived in our first house, I pushed the girls on the nearby park swings, going ever higher, as they screamed, "Push me around the bar, Daddy!" In summer, we went tubing; in winter, we went sledding. When feasible, we ate outdoors and listened to the crickets until the mosquitoes drove us inside. At night, Daisy and I read to the children. We

recited with them the Jewish prayer, the Shema Yisrael. I tucked
them in and sang their favorite tune, "I see the moon, the moon
sees me," in my totally out-of-tune voice. These were extremely busy,
happy years. Life in Minnesota was good for our family.

Our fourth daughter, Dana Alexandra, was born on December
26, 1968. With four children, we outgrew our two-bedroom rented
house. In 1969 we purchased a home large enough for all of us on
a small lake. Here our children grew up, went to various schools in
the Twin Cities, and emerged as adults. Daisy and I still live com-
fortably in this house, enjoy the seasons in the morning light and
watch the moon at night from our bedroom.

I did my best to spend time with my children during these for-
mative years. I rarely, if ever, missed any of their athletic events,
debate contests, or assemblies. I often slipped into the stands of an
event straight from the hospital and sat down next to Daisy, who
handed me my dinner sandwich. When I came home at night,
Buck, our German shepherd, greeted me with an exuberant charge.

The children went to various colleges and graduate schools.
They became a lawyer and humane education advocate, a medical
writer and editor, a communications expert and children's book
writer, and an actor and scriptwriter. Three of them chose to marry:
a statistician, a linguist and translator, and an actor and disabili-
ties advocate joined our family. Three of them live in Minnesota
or neighboring Wisconsin. Not only have Daisy and I lived two-
thirds of our lives in Minnesota, but our children and their families
share our preference for the Midwest. Over the years, we have been
blessed with six wonderful grandchildren, four girls and two boys.
Two are out in the world, three are in college, and one fledgling is
still at home.

Daisy taught literature at the University of Minnesota until she
completed her PhD in 1971 at the university. She published four
award-winning books for young readers and an award-winning

book of poetry. She taught a course in writing for children at the
University of Minnesota College of Continuing Education for
Women, and courses in poetry at the Loft Literary Center. In 1980,
in partnership with visual artist R. W. Scholes, she started *The Milkweed Chronicle,* a journal dedicated to a collaboration of words and
images. In 1984, this publication morphed into Milkweed Editions
and became a leading national, independent, not-for-profit press.
With more than a million copies in print, Daisy retired as publisher and editor in chief of Milkweed Editions in 2003. In 2006 she
founded The Gryphon Press, publishing children's picture books
about the human–animal bond, each book with a message about
animal well-being. Awards recognizing her contributions include
the McKnight Distinguished Artist Award, the Kay Sexton Award,
an honorary doctor of humane letters from the University of Minnesota, and the National Book Critics Circle Ivan Sandrof Lifetime
Achievement Award, a prize rarely given to individuals outside the
trade cities of New York and Los Angeles.

———

When I started my clinical career, I was a true general surgeon—I
operated in the abdomen, the chest, the head and neck, and the
extremities. As all of us in surgery were forced into specialization,
I became a gastrointestinal surgeon, from esophagus to colon,
including hernias. By the time esophageal and colorectal surgery
also became specialties, I too was a specialist—a bariatric or obesity surgeon, a vocation dedicated not only to certain operations
but to the lifelong care of the patient. Dr. Robert Goodale, Dr.
Jack Delaney, and I were among the first to perform laparoscopic
surgery at the University of Minnesota, mostly cholecystectomies.
When the younger generation, primarily schooled in this technique, entered clinical practice, I concentrated on procedures as yet

in the open surgery domain, focusing on the bariatric operation of duodenal switch and revisions of prior bariatric procedures.

As a clinician and technical surgeon, I wanted to be as good as Varco. I never took an operation for granted. I never believed that there was minor and major surgery; there were only minor and major surgeons. Before each case, regardless of how many times I had previously performed the procedure, I rehearsed it in my mind. I entered the operating room with a game plan but prepared to deviate from it as necessary. I discontinued my clinical practice at the age of eighty-two; while I have not missed the telephone calls at night, I do miss seeing patients, and I continuously long for the sanctuary, the home away from home, of the operating room. I have performed well over ten thousand operations in my lifetime, and I like to believe that they were beneficial, perhaps even life-changing for the better for my patients. A good friend, the late Monsignor Terrence Murphy, a renowned educator and president of the University of St. Thomas, responded to my question of how he would like to be remembered by saying that he hoped people would say, "He was a good priest." I empathize with his aspiration. I hope people will say about me, "He was a good surgeon."

As a teacher, I have instructed surgical residents and medical and engineering students for more than fifty years. Over time, I have enjoyed working with close to one hundred surgical residents and fellows, engineering majors, and undergraduates in my laboratory. Many have gone on to brilliant careers, including Marshall Schwartz, distinguished pediatric surgeon, department chair and former Regent of the American College of Surgeons; Perry J. Blackshear, a Howard Hughes Lifetime Medical Fellow; and Peter Agre, Nobel Laureate in chemistry. My love for teaching has elicited invitations to many conferences in cities around the world, opportunities to meet experts and confer with them in my fields of interest.

Writing about my work is a craft I thoroughly enjoy. I have published eleven books as author or editor, eighty book chapters, and 350 papers in the peer-reviewed medical literature. For the past three years, I have written a column for *General Surgery News* that gives me the privilege of reaching fellow surgeons in a popular journal, as well as the opportunity to have a bully pulpit to vent my views of, grievances about, and aspirations for the discipline of surgery.

Over the years, my research has been concentrated in hypercholesterolemia and atherosclerosis, medical engineering, and metabolic/bariatric surgery.

None of the early lipid/atherosclerosis trials, funded and advocated by the National Heart, Lung and Blood Institute (NHLBI) of the National Institutes of Health (NIH), utilized robust lipid-lowering modalities, and all proved to be negative or inconclusive. In 1973, Richard Varco and I proposed to the NHLBI the Program on the Surgical Control of the Hyperlipidemias (POSCH) study, which was to employ as the lipid-lowering agent the partial ileal bypass (PIB) operation, our 1960s introduction into cholesterol-lowering therapeutics. After several site visits and numerous tribulations, POSCH was funded. It eventually cost $60 million, the largest investigator-initiated grant (in contrast to an NIH-initiated contract) in the history of the NIH at that time.

POSCH was conducted in four geographically distributed clinics. Between 1975 and 1983, after recruitment, screening, and obtaining informed consent, the study randomized 838 survivors of a single myocardial infarction (heart attack) to cholesterol lowering with diet instruction only (417 patients in the control group) and to diet instruction plus PIB (421 patients in the intervention group).

In October 1990, at the American College of Surgeons annual meeting in San Francisco, POSCH was provided with an extended time slot to present the study findings. Concurrently, the results were published in the *New England Journal of Medicine* and nationally distributed in the media by the *New York Times*.

POSCH was the first definitive study to prove the lipid/atherosclerosis hypothesis, and the first and only to use surgery for the intervention modality. With high statistical significance, POSCH demonstrated that the PIB-intervention group, in comparison to the control group, sustained a 35 percent reduction in the combined end point of atherosclerotic death or a new myocardial infarction, a 14.6 percent difference in the development of peripheral vascular disease, and a 16.1 percent reduction in the need for heart surgery. Over time, there was an increase in life expectancy in the PIB group that was sustained for more than thirty-five years of follow-up. Uniquely, POSCH included a trial within the trial by following sequential changes in coronary atherosclerosis in arteriograms performed at 0, 3, 5, 7, and 10 years. The arteriographic study not only demonstrated the retardation of progression of atherosclerosis in the PIB group, but, for the first time, actual coronary artery plaque regression.

Comparable to my unpleasant experience with Louis Katz at the introduction of the PIB, an element of the nonsurgical medical community violently opposed surgical therapy, a possibly curative therapy, for what they considered a medical problem. My opponent this time was not an individual but an institution—the NHLBI. At every turn, the NHLBI project officer, whose official role it was to support the study to which he was assigned, opposed it, even speaking out publicly against POSCH funding at a program review in Bethesda. Fortunately, the concept was supported by the majority of the prominent site visitors of the multiple POSCH peer reviews, as well as the eminent non-NHLBI members of the POSCH Data Monitoring Committee and Policy Advisory Board.

I have found it difficult to ascertain the motive for the NHLBI opposition. Was it the result of an antisurgery sentiment by the

NHLBI? Was it related to favoring a statin drug trial, published two years after the POSCH results were made public, which had been performed on an NHLBI contract, and for which the NHLBI had received $10 million from industry?

In addition to surgery, I have had a career in biomedical engineering. My entry into the field of biomedical engineering emanated from my belief that an understanding of engineering principles should be taught in medical school. To understand the human body, in health and in disease, the medical school curriculum dissects coordinated functions into their component basic source aspects. Thus, to study cardiovascular actions, we separately analyze gross and microscopic heart and vessel anatomy, the physiology of muscle contraction, and the biochemistry of impulse transmission. Why not, I thought, the rheology of blood flow as well? To investigate this subject, I posed to a friend and colleague, Perry L. Blackshear Jr., chair of mechanical engineering and father of Perry J. Blackshear, the question of why atherosclerotic plaques form at the bend of an arterial bifurcation. He came back with a long series of equations when we next met for lunch, demonstrating that the engineering mechanics for plaques to form within the vessel wall favored the area opposite to a bend in an artery. I told him that this site based on his equations differed from reality by 180 degrees. He smiled and said, "No problem: change all the pluses in the equation to minuses and vice versa, and we'll have it right." This moment of mirth laid the foundation for our efforts to build a Department of Biomedical Engineering and to introduce biomedical engineering into medical school curricula.

To begin this venture, Perry and I enlisted the help of Dr. Richard Varco, Dr. Demetre Nicoloff, and Dr. Kenneth Keller, chair of chemical engineering and future president of the university. Our concept was accepted by the medical school and we were designated the Faculty of Biomedical Engineering. We were not a department, because we were given no independent funding. Several years later, because we now had master's degree and PhD candidates, the university was obligated to provide us departmental status. From this small nucleus, the Department of Biomedical Engineering has become one of the largest departments at the University of Minnesota, with its own building and several ancillary facilities around the university complex.

At first, I incorporated engineering research into my surgery lipid laboratory. As our engineering projects acquired independent funding, I acquired a second laboratory in the mechanical engineering building. We set out to provide useful instrumentation that would improve patient care and explore new vistas in medical device utilization. The products of our bioengineering research included the first and the second versions of implantable infusion pumps, multiple one-way and two-way catheters, a peritoneal shunt to treat ascites (peritoneal fluid accumulation secondary to liver failure), an oxygen transport analyzer, and an expandable platform to facilitate abdominal or perirectal surgery. The ubiquitous implantable infusion port, an offshoot of our pump technology, for a plethora of therapeutics was a product of the laboratory as well. We were persuaded, foolishly on our part, not to patent this device, allowing several companies to profit in the millions of dollars with no return to our group or to the University of Minnesota.

The implantable pumps have been and can be used for infusion of heparin, analgesics and antispasmodics, chemotherapeutic agents, and insulin. We employed our first-generation pump to deliver heparin intravenously to individuals in need of acute anticoagulation but refractory to the standard subcutaneous administration of this agent. Subsequent to our original publication on our implantable infusion pump and the market availability of the device by the Infusaid Corporation, the Mayo Clinic started using this device for intraspinal column injections of agents for the control of chronic pain and spastitivity, allowing previously neurologically incapacitated patients to live active lives.

We were the first to use our implantable pump for the administration of chemotherapeutic drugs directly to the liver by the portal vein, which exclusively flows to the liver, to treat metastatic cancer liver implants, allowing for delivery of up to five hundred-fold the concentration of the drug directly to the tumor. Subsequently, the Memorial Sloan Kettering Cancer Center in New York City, one of the premium cancer centers in the nation, began a major program for the treatment of liver metastases with the use of our implantable pump.

The most promising use of the implantable infusion pump is in the management of type 2 diabetes. External insulin pumps were postulated as early as the 1960s; we preceded their utilization with our totally implantable pump. In 1982, our group published in the *New England Journal of Medicine* our report of one year of successful pump delivery of insulin therapy in five patients.

The utility of the implantable infusion pump for the therapy of type 2 diabetes led to the formation of the International Study Group on Implantable Insulin Delivery Devices (ISGIID) on the impetus of Dr. Karl Irsigler, a Viennese diabetologist, and Dr. Attila Szabo, head of European markets for the insulin manufacturer Novo. ISGIID flourished for about ten years based on reports of several hundred pump implantations for insulin delivery in patients with type 2 diabetes. Unfortunately, the implantable pump for insulin delivery to patients with diabetes has not, to date, matured, for lack of a reliable implantable glucose sensor to regulate pump outflow.

Our catheters allowed for intravenous infusions without backflow. Our peritoneal shunt provided a mechanism for active, as well as passive, pumping of ascitic fluid into the chest cavity for reabsorption. Our oxygen transport analyzer, the only such available device, can be used for many purposes, including separating donated blood in blood banks and in the military for fast oxygen utilization by the recipient following acute trauma, as well as regular oxygen availability for patients with chronic blood loss.

Our operative platform invention consists of a small port of entry into the abdominal cavity or per rectum, with the ability to open mechanically blades lit to expose the area of interest within the abdomen or colon. The use of this device avoids general anesthesia, tracheal intubation, and gaseous insufflation for visualization, thereby making the operation feasible under local and sedation anesthesia, with less patient discomfort, earlier hospital discharge, and increased safety.

Since Richard Varco forced my entry into the discipline of bariatric surgery in 1966, I have become known primarily for my work in this field. I have proffered innovations to the operative procedures used in bariatric surgery, been an outspoken advocate for and historian of the field, added to its literature, and served in leadership roles for the field's major organizations. I believe that my main contribution to this specialty has been presenting the evidence that bariatric surgery is a part of the emerging discipline of metabolic surgery.

In *Metabolic Surgery*, a book published in 1987, Richard Varco and I defined metabolic surgery as "the operative manipulation of a normal organ or organ system to achieve a biological result for a potential health gain." Traditionally, surgery has concentrated on organs gone bad—organs diseased, injured, or malfunctioning. In contrast, metabolic surgery focuses on altering normal organs with the intent of effecting change in the body's internal milieu. This perception expresses a more holistic approach to disease, considering a disease not as representing an error in a specific organ but, rather, as having a complex metabolic mosaic of causation.

Metabolic surgery is not new. More than 120 years ago,

physicians found that the removal of normal ovaries would cause the retardation of breast cancer metastases. Several other metabolic surgery procedures became popular during the twentieth century. Probably the most commonly performed metabolic surgery prior to the introduction of bariatric surgery was surgery for peptic ulcer disease. This surgery involved the resection of various segments of normal stomach and the division of branches of normal vagus nerves in order to cure a duodenal ulcer that remained, except for emergencies, untouched by the hand of the surgeon. The partial ileal bypass for hyperlipidemia, and its utilization in the POSCH trial, was metabolic surgery. Extension of the concept of metabolic surgery represents a major future opportunity for the practice of surgery.

Meta-analysis is the powerful statistical tool of combining the results of multiple scientific studies to derive a common truth. It is considered the apex of the universally cited evidence-based pyramid of scientific knowledge. In 2004, with the help of my longtime administrative assistant, Danette Oien, coworkers and I published the first meta-analysis of the powerful affirmative effects of the four popular bariatric operations of the time (gastric banding, vertical banded gastroplasty, gastric bypass, and biliopancreatic diversion/ duodenal switch) on weight loss and on the metabolic diseases of type 2 diabetes, hyperlipidemia, and hypertension. This paper firmly established the credentials of bariatric surgery as metabolic surgery, that is, operating on putatively normal organs to establish a metabolic effect.

In 2009, our group published a meta-analysis dedicated solely to the mitigation of type 2 diabetes by bariatric surgery procedures. This paper served as an impetus for the current worldwide search for metabolic surgery operations for the treatment of type 2 diabetes, with or without weight loss, in and out of the abdominal cavity. It may also have been the stimulus for the long-overdue recognition of obesity as a disease by the American Medical Association (AMA) and for the recommendation by the American Diabetes Association (ADA) that metabolic/bariatric surgery be included in the armamentarium of type 2 diabetes therapies.

Within the field of surgery, various societies have recognized the vital addition of metabolic surgery to their discipline by changing their names. The American Society for Bariatric Surgery became the American Society for Metabolic and Bariatric Surgery (ASMBS), and the International Federation for the Surgery of Obesity became the International Federation for the Surgery of Obesity and Metabolic Disorders (IFSO). In 2018, the American College of Surgery (ACS) asked me to host a symposium on the promise of metabolic surgery. The papers generated by the symposium were published in seven consecutive issues of the *ACS College Bulletin*. Essentially, all meetings and publications on surgical management of obesity now refer to the operative procedures as metabolic/bariatric surgery or simply as metabolic surgery. In 2019, the ACS honored me for my work in metabolic surgery with the Jacobson Innovation Award for "groundbreaking surgical development or technique."

Interestingly, at times old data find new meaning. Recently, we have ascertained that the control group in the POSCH trial had a 2.7-fold higher incidence of type 2 diabetes over thirty years of follow-up than that exhibited by the PIB-intervention group. We are assessing the PIB operation as possibly having an even greater therapeutic potential than its cholesterol-lowering effect.

I am currently occupied with several projects, including working with the American College of Surgeons to actualize the concept of metabolic surgery; and working with the National Football League Players Association, and its affiliate, the Living Heart Foundation–Heart Obesity Prevention Education program, to increase public awareness of the problems of obesity and diabetes and acknowledge the poorly recognized association of neurocognitive impairment (e.g., early dementia and Alzheimer's) with obesity.

In my lifetime, academic surgery has been and remains for me a source of never-ending challenges and opportunities to learn, to invent, to experiment, and to engage with remarkable colleagues. I still find it worthwhile to continue this journey. In my long career, the great reward has always been the joy of the process itself—the surgery, the teaching, the research. The promise of finding new and better outcomes for patients is a constant inspiration; the work is always fresh and can never be concluded.

As the longest-serving member of the University of Minnesota Department of Surgery, I am the only current faculty member from the Wangensteen era. As a chronicler of that era, I cherish the fact that I served as the first Owen H. and Sarah Davidson Wangensteen Chair in Experimental Surgery. So many of my colleagues participated in, contributed to, and believed in the unique world of our Department of Surgery. The world to which we were privileged to belong was the dream of one of the greatest medical dreamers of the twentieth century, Dr. Owen H. Wangensteen. His personal era ended with his retirement in 1967; however, his dream became reality.

Acknowledgments

There could not be a better editor than Erik Anderson, who guided me through the construction and the process of revising this book. He was enthusiastic about its contents and believed in its approach. We worked well and harmoniously to achieve the final result. The members of the staff of the University of Minnesota Press, led by director Douglas Armato, were generous with their time and expertise. Thanks to Daniel Ochsner for his excellent production work.

My wife, Daisy Emilie Buchwald, author, editor, and publisher in her own right, served as my substantive editor, reading every word several times. She kept me on track, prevented foolish commentary, and separated substance from trivia.

Danette Oien word-processed the manuscript in all of its iterations, making corrections and revisions with patience and understanding as a most appreciated gift to me. I am grateful for her friendship.

Thanks to Mary Knatterud, professional writer and editor, for her editorial comments.

I thank Christine Johnson, my personal assistant, for handling the book's affiliated correspondence.

I appreciate the assistance of Jerry Vincent, Department of Surgery; Lois Hendrickson, chief librarian, Wangensteen Historical Library; and Erik Moore, University Archives and Elmer L. Andersen Library, for their time and for providing me with visual and historical materials.

Index

All locations in Minnesota unless otherwise specified.

Agre, Peter (MD), 107, 173
Alden, John F. (MD), 164
American College of Surgeons,
  Surgical Forum, Wangensteen's
  origination of, 23
American Heart Association (AHA):
  Established Investigator Award,
  103–4, 127; HB's presentation to,
  99–100, 101
Amplatz, Kurt (MD), 168
Anderson, Ron and Bev (Edina
  neighbors), 39
Anoka State Hospital, HB's rotation
  at, 52, 53–55, 59–61, 129
Anthony, Susan B., quote from, 52
anticlotting agents, introduction
  of, 166. *See also* liver surgeries/
  transplants; open-heart surgery
Apgar, Virginia (MD), 65
atherosclerotic cardiovascular
  disease, 95–100, 108. *See also* lipid/
  atherosclerosis research
Aust, J. (Joseph) Bradley (MD), 49,
  52, 80, 87–88, 154; HB's rebellion
  against, 143–44, 145, 151; White

Surgery service reporting to,
  40–41, 44–45, 46, 47, 122–23

Bakken, Earl, 28
bariatric (obesity) surgery, 26,
  138, 163, 172, 180–82. *See also*
  metabolic/bariatric surgery
Barnard, Christiaan (MD), 22
Bear, Richard S. (Dean), HB's
  meeting with, 103
Bertish, Josephine, 106, 152
bile acids, 95–96
bile salt, absorption of, 108
biochemistry, HB's MS in. *See*
  Buchwald, HB, MS and PhD
  degrees
biomedical engineering, 175–77
Blackshear, Perry J. (MD), 173, 176
Bloch, Jack (MD), 110, 111, 154–55;
  HB's friendship with, 14, 48,
  62–63, 115, 125, 152; residency at U
  of M, 40–41, 44, 47
Blue Surgery service, 35, 46; HB's
  rotation on, 118
Boruski, Mary "Mamie," 40

Boundary Waters Canoe Area
Wilderness, 69
bowel anastomoses, 149
bowel obstruction, 20–21, 163
breast cancer, radical mastectomies
for, 41–42
bubble pump oxygenator, invention
of, 26, 28
Buchwald, Amy Elizabeth (daughter
of HB), 114–15, 132, 141; birth of,
64, 65–66, 91
Buchwald, Andor (father of HB),
7–8, 10, 141
Buchwald, Claire Gretchen (PhD)
(daughter of HB), 141
Buchwald, Daisy Emilie Bix (PhD)
(wife of HB): career, 13, 40, 64,
171–72; childbirth experiences,
64–66, 115–16, 141; MA and PhD
degrees, 13, 40, 64, 112–13, 171;
marriage to HB, 11–12, 13; move to
Minneapolis, 1, 15–16, 34; musical
interests, 37
Buchwald, Dana Alexandra (JD)
(daughter of HB), 171
Buchwald, Henry (MD) (HB), 151,
182; additional jobs during
residency, 78–79, 102; assistant
professorship, 144–45, 146–52;
birth and childhood, 5, 9–10;
chief residency, 133–45, 147;
education, 3, 10–11; English Ford
Popular automobile, 1, 66–67;
family life, 170–71; internship,
12–13, 14, 15, 44; marriage to Daisy,
11–12, 13; military service, 1–3,

34–35, 54; move to Minneapolis,
1, 15–16, 34; MS and PhD degrees,
14, 80, 92–93, 101–2, 109–13, 147–50;
publications, 173–74; surgical
specialty, 15, 54–55, 80. See also
laboratories, HB's; research, HB's;
and under individual surgical
services
Buchwald, Jane (daughter of HB), 1,
15–16, 34, 64–65, 91, 141
Buchwald, Renée (mother of HB),
8, 9, 141
Byers, Sanford O. (PhD), 96

cancer: breast, 41–42; pediatric cancer
surgeries, 166–67; second-look
procedure, 71–72; skin, 77
cardiac catheterization procedure,
28, 167
cardiac pacemakers and valve
prostheses, 28, 156
cardiovascular surgery, 82, 129–30,
156, 167. See also atherosclerotic
cardiovascular disease; heart
surgery/transplants; open-heart
surgery
Castaneda, Aldo (MD), 90, 136, 147,
148–49, 151, 152, 167
Cerra, Frank (MD), 168
Chief, The. See Wangensteen, Owen
Harding (MD)
cholesterol: absorption of, 97, 99,
107–8; lowering, 95–100, 109,
174–75
cholesterol/atherosclerosis
hypothesis, 108

chronic wasting disease, 69
Cicero, Marcus Tullius, quote from,
    146
Coffman, Lotus Delta (Dean), 23
Cohen, Morley (MD), 29
Columbia-Presbyterian Medical
    Center (New York, New York),
    HB's internship at, 14, 15, 44
Columbia University, College of
    Physicians and Surgeons (P&S,
    New York, New York), HB
    Buchwald's education at, 3, 11–12
concentration camps, Nazi, 5–7
Cooley, Denton (MD), 69, 70
Corelli, Franco, 79
Cournand, Andre (MD), 167
Curtis Hotel (Minneapolis), 34

DeBakey, Michael E. (MD), 70–71
Delaney, John P. "Jack" (MD), 125–28,
    129, 152, 155, 172
DeWall, Richard (MD), 26, 28
diabetes, type 2, 178, 180–82
Diehl, Harold S. (Dean), 20
Dragstedt, Lester R. (MD), 69, 70
Dudrick, Stanley J. (MD), 168
dumping syndrome, HB's research
    into, 76
Dunphy, J. Englebert (MD), 69, 70

East Coast medical schools, 5,
    30–32, 33, 37, 47, 49–50. See also
    Columbia-Presbyterian Medical
    Center (New York, New York),
    HB's internship at
Edina, Buchwalds' home in, 36, 37–38

Eichmann, Adolf, annihilation of
    Jews, 6
Eiseman, Benjamin "Ben" (MD), 165
Ellis, Cassius (MD), 151
Ellison, Robert G. (MD), 69–70
enterohepatic bile acid/cholesterol
    cycle, 95–96

fecal transplantation, 164–65
Fitch, Laurie (PhD), 106, 152
Frantz, Ivan D. (MD), 93, 111
Friedman, Meyer (MD), 96
Frykman, Howard (MD), 149

Gans, Henry (MD), 166
gastric bypass surgery, 164. See also
    bariatric (obesity) surgery;
    metabolic/bariatric surgery
gastric cooling/freezing, research
    into, 77–78
gastrointestinal surgery, 21, 118, 129,
    164–65, 166; HB's specialization
    in, 95, 130, 147, 172. See also
    bariatric (obesity) surgery;
    metabolic/bariatric surgery;
    pancreas transplants; partial ileal
    bypass surgery
Gebhard, Roger (MD), 106, 152
Ge Hong (holistic medicine
    practitioner), 165
Goldberg, Stanley (MD), 149
Goodale, Robert "Bob" (MD), 128–29,
    157, 172
Grage, Theodor (MD), 47, 48–49,
    122–23, 157
grand rounds, 49–51, 160–61

Green Surgery service, 28, 35, 45–46
Griffen, Ward, Jr. (MD), 71, 117, 136,
    137, 147, 152, 164
Gross, Robert E. (MD), 69, 70
Gryphon Press (Minneapolis), 172
Gueron, Moshe (MD), 28
Gunning, Marlise N., 96

Harken, Dwight (MD), 12
Haskell, Bennie and Fritzi, 123
heart-lung machine, 28
heart surgery/transplants, 22, 46, 175.
    See also cardiovascular surgery;
    open-heart surgery
hemicorporectomy surgery, 41
Hitler, Adolf, annihilation of Jews, 6
Howell, James, quote from, 62
Humphrey, Edward (MD), 129
Humphrey, Hubert H., quote from,
    125
Humphreys, George H., II (MD), 14
hyperlipidemias, 99. See also partial
    ileal bypass surgery; Program
    on the Surgical Control of the
    Hyperlipidemias (POSCH)
hypnosis, for pain control, 73–74

implantable pumps, 177–78
intensive-care units, 168
International Study Group on
    Implantable Insulin Delivery
    Devices (ISGIID), 178
intestinal obstructions, 20–21, 163
intestine transplants, 157
inventions, 20–21, 26, 28, 157, 163,
    177–78, 179

Irsigler, Karl (MD), 178
Ito, Chikashi (MD), 164

Jacobson Innovation Award, 181
jejunoileal bypass surgery, 138
Jews, annihilation of, 6–7
Josephsons (Edina neighbors), 39–40

Katz, Louis (MD), attack on HB's
    research, 99–100, 101, 103, 108, 175
Keller, Kenneth (PhD), 176–77
Kennedy, Byrl James "B. J." (MD), 128
kidney transplants, 30, 120
Kremen, Arnold (MD), 29, 138, 150–51

laboratories, HB's, 91–109; acquiring,
    91–94, 151–52, 177; fellows working
    in, 105–7, 173; funding, 102–4,
    108–9, 127; Varco's support for, 135.
    See also research, HB's
Lack, Leon, 96
laparoscopic surgery, 129, 172
Leonard, Arnold S. "Arny" (MD), 131,
    166
Levy, Morris (MD), 28
Lewis, F. John (MD), 25–26
Lillehei, Clarence Walton "Walt"
    (MD), 30, 32, 103, 168; clash with
    Najarian, 155–56. 157; Green
    Surgery service reporting to,
    27–29, 35, 45–46; move to Cornell
    Medical School, 130, 154; open-
    heart surgery, 25–26, 27, 82, 168
Lillehei, Richard Carlton "Rich"
    (MD), 27, 29–30, 32, 152; and
    dedicated intensive-care units,

168; Najarian's relationship with, 156–57; and Red Surgery service, 46, 118–22, 134; Varco's relationship with, 134–35, 136
Linner, John (MD), jejunoileal bypass surgery, 138
lipid/atherosclerosis research, 138–39, 174–75. *See also* atherosclerotic cardiovascular disease
Lister, Joseph (MD), 20, 21
liver surgeries/transplants, 70–71, 166, 176, 178
Lyon, Elias P. (Dean), 19, 23

Mary Imogene Bassett Hospital (Cooperstown, New York), HB's externship at, 14–15
Mason, Edward E. (MD), 164
Mayo, William J. (MD), 18, 23
Mayo Clinic (Rochester), 4, 18, 167, 177–78
McFee, Arthur (MD), 154
McQuarrie, Donald G. "Don" (MD), 52, 54, 62, 129, 152
Memorial Sloan Kettering Cancer Center (New York, New York), 178
Meredith, Char, quote from, 82
meta-analysis, use of, 180–81
metabolic/bariatric surgery, 95, 163–64, 179–80. *See also* bariatric (obesity) surgery; partial ileal bypass surgery
microassay apparatus, 46–47
military service: HB's, 1–3, 34–35, 54; value of, 125, 154, 164

Milkweed Editions (Minneapolis), 172
Milliken, Bill, quote from, 82
Minneapolis: anti-Semitism in, 9, 36, 37, 39; Buchwald family's move to, 1, 15–16, 34. *See also* Edina, Buchwalds' home in
Moberg, Allen (MD), 119
Mohs's paste surgery, 77
Monk, Samuel, 40
Montaigne, Michel de, quote from, 117
Moore, Francis "Franny" (MD), 12–13
Moore, George E. (MD), 150
Moore, Richard "Dick" (MD), 109
Mt. Sinai Hospital (Minneapolis), 37, 150–51
Murphy, Terrence (Mgsr.), 173
Murray, Joseph E. (MD), 120–21
myocardial infarctions, 108

Najarian, John (MD): chair of U of M Department of Surgery, 123, 127, 129, 130, 153, 160–61; Walt Lillehei's clash with, 155–56, 157
Nakayama, Komei (MD), 70
Nicoloff, Demetre "Nick" (MD), 129–30, 176–77

obesity. *See* bariatric (obesity) surgery
Oien, Danette, 180
open-heart surgery, 28, 166, 168; first successful, 25–26, 27. *See also* cardiovascular surgery; heart surgery/transplants

operative platform invention, 179
Orange Surgery service, 35, 46; HB's
    rotations on, 80, 82–91, 99, 135–41
Osler, William (MD), quote from, 1
oxygen transport analyzer, 179

pancreas transplants, 30, 118, 157,
    163–63
pancreatic sphincter of Oddi surgery,
    127
Papermaster, Ralph (DDS), 73
parenteral nutrition, 168
partial ileal bypass surgery: HB's
    performance of, 135, 138; in
    juvenile animals, 107; lowering
    cholesterol through, 95–101,
    174–75; research on, 95–101, 107–9,
    147–50; results of, 108, 109, 117,
    175. See also metabolic/bariatric
    surgery; Program on the Surgical
    Control of the Hyperlipidemias
    (POSCH)
patent ductus arteriosus (PDA)
    repair, 83
patient care, 87, 130; East Coast
    tradition, 31–32; HB's approach
    to, 55, 59–60, 91, 172; innovations
    in, 75, 95, 118–19, 177; intensive
    care units, 168
pediatric surgeries, 107, 131, 132, 166
peptic ulcer surgery, 180
peritoneal shunts, 178–79
Pernkopf, Edward (Prof.), anatomical
    atlas, 90
Perry, John F. (MD), 46, 52, 118
PhD degrees, 22, 162. See also

Buchwald, Daisy Emilie Bix
    (PhD) (wife of HB), MA and PhD
    degrees; Buchwald, Henry (MD),
    MS and PhD degrees
Phillips, Jay, 37
Plummer, Henry S. (MD), 18
Powers, John H. (MD), 14
Prem, Konald (MD), 65, 66, 115, 146–47
Printen, Kenneth J. (MD), 164
Program on the Surgical Control of
    the Hyperlipidemias (POSCH),
    106, 135, 174–76, 180, 181. See also
    partial ileal bypass surgery
Purple Surgery service, 35; HB's
    rotations on, 62–64, 67–74, 75–80,
    117, 129, 141–45, 165

Quervain, Fritz de (MD), 19

Red Surgery service, 35, 46, 126; HB's
    rotation on, 118–22, 133–34
research: combining with surgery
    and scholarship, 61, 156, 169, 170,
    182; incorporating into residency
    program, 3, 4, 5, 15, 20–23, 25, 162;
    translational, 95
research, HB's, 75–78; in
    bioengineering, 176–77; on
    lipid/atherosclerosis, 100, 138–39,
    174–75; on partial ileal bypass
    surgery, 95–101, 107–9, 147–50. See
    also laboratories, HB's
residency program. See research,
    incorporating into residency pro-
    gram; University of Minnesota
    (U of M, Minneapolis) Medical

School, residency program;
Wangensteen, Owen Harding
(MD), surgical residency program
designed by
Richards, Dickinson (MD), 167
Root, Harlan (MD), 154

Sagan, Carl, quote from, 105
Saltzmann, Daniel (MD), 132
Samuel D. Gross Prize, 150, 161
Schwartz, Marshall (MD), 106–7, 152,
173
Semmelweis, Ignaz (MD), 20, 21
serum histamine, measuring, 46–47
Shumway, Norman (MD), 22
Society of University Surgeons,
Wangensteen's founding of, 23
Sones, F. Mason (MD), 167
Speakes, George, 38–39
Stammon, Richard E. (Dean), 22
Starzl, Thomas E. (MD), 69, 70
Steer, Charles (MD), 65
Stillwater State Prison, HB's rotation
at, 52, 55–61
Strachauer, Arthur (MD), 18, 19
Sullivan, W. Albert (MD), 47–48,
123–24, 152
surgery: academic, 44, 150, 153, 169,
182; combining research and
scholarship with, 61, 156, 169,
170, 182. See also University
of Minnesota (U of M,
Minneapolis) Department of
Surgery; and specific types of
surgeries and surgical services
designated by color

Surgery (journal), Wangensteen's
founding of, 23
Szabo, Attila (PhD), 178

Talmud, The, quote from, 170
Tebaldi, Renata, 79
Thal, Alan (MD), 46–47, 118
tracheal stimulation, postoperative
use of, 78
transplant surgeries, 153, 157, 163.
See also fecal transplantation;
heart surgery/transplants; kidney
transplants; liver surgeries/
transplants; pancreas transplants
Tucker, Richard, 79
Tuna, Naip (MD), 119, 141

University of Minnesota Physicians
(UMP), 127, 131
University of Minnesota
(Minneapolis) (U of M)
Department of Biomedical
Engineering, 176–77
University of Minnesota
(Minneapolis) (U of M)
Department of Surgery, 37,
182; accomplishments, 153–54,
163–69; decorum and permissible
behavior, 119–20; grand rounds,
50–51; system of, 32–33, 35, 44–51;
Wangensteen (MD) in charge of,
19–24, 32–33, 61
University of Minnesota
(Minneapolis) (U of M) Medical
School: accomplishments of
graduates from, 163–69; residency

program, 34–37, 44–51, 61, 64, 92–93, 170. *See also* Wangensteen, Owen Harding (MD), surgical residence program designed by

Varco, Richard L. (MD), 24–27, 30, 32, 103, 107, 127, 156; awards, 26, 29; bariatric (obesity) surgery, 163–64, 179; and dedicated intensive-care units, 168; disciples of, 129–30; HB's friendship with, 139–41, 146–47; introducing biomedical engineering into medical school, 176–77; jejunoileal bypass surgery, 138; mentoring HB, 152, 173; Orange Surgery service reporting to, 35, 46, 80, 82–91, 99, 135–41; participating in grand rounds, 51; pediatric cardiovascular surgery, 166; research space supervised by, 93, 94, 135; retirement, 130, 135–36, 158–60; Richard Lillehei's relationship with, 134–35, 136; treatment of Amy Buchwald, 66, 91. *See also* Program on the Surgical Control of the Hyperlipidemias (POSCH)
vitamin B12, absorption of, 108
Voyageurs National Park (International Falls), 69

Wangensteen, Owen Harding (MD): accomplishments, 20–21, 23, 163; biographical information, 4–5, 17–20; chair of U of M Department of Surgery, 19–24, 32–33, 61; and HB's laboratory funding, 103–4; honors, 150, 160–61; laboratory, 126; lymph node resection on Clarence Lillehei, 29; mentoring HB, 100–101, 152; participating in grand rounds, 51; philosophy of surgery, 25, 155; placing graduates outside Minnesota, 150–51; Purple Surgery service reporting to, 35, 62–64, 68–74, 75–80, 117, 141–45, 165; quotes from, 17, 44, 75, 92, 133, 153; retirement, 141–42, 153, 160–62; surgical residency program designed by, 3–5, 21–24, 64, 79–80, 163, 168, 169–70
Wangensteen, Sarah Davidson (wife of Owen), 23–24, 161–62
Wangensteen suction, 20–21, 163
Warden, Herbert (MD), 29
Weckwerth, Vernon (PhD), 101
Weiner, I. M. (PhD), 96
Whipple surgery, 137
White Surgery service, 46, 47; HB's rotations on, 35, 40–45, 54, 122–24
Whitney Foundation, laboratory funding from, 103
Wiesel, Elie, quote from, 34
World War II, 6–7

Zollinger, Robert M. (MD), 69–70

HENRY BUCHWALD is professor of surgery and biomedical engineering and the Owen H. and Sarah Davidson Wangensteen Chair in Experimental Surgery Emeritus at the University of Minnesota. He holds nineteen patents for medical devices, including the first implantable infusion pump. He received the University of Minnesota Diehl Award and was elected to membership in the University of Minnesota Academic Health Center's Academy for Excellence in Health Research in 2015. In 2019 he was awarded the American College of Surgery Jacobson Innovation Award for lifetime achievement in research and scholarship, and in 2020 the Gold Medal for Outstanding Achievement in Medical Research by the Columbia University Vagelos College of Physicians and Surgeons. He is an honorary member of the Royal College of Surgeons in England and past president of five surgical organizations. He and his wife, Emilie Buchwald, live in Minneapolis.